Fat Oppression and Psychotherapy: A Feminist Perspective

Fat Oppression and Psychotherapy: A Feminist Perspective

Laura S. Brown, PhD
Esther D. Rothblum, PhD
Editors

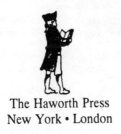

The Haworth Press
New York • London

Fat Oppression and Psychotherapy: A Feminist Perspective has also been published as *Women & Therapy*, Volume 8, Number 3 1989.

The Haworth Press, Inc. 10 Alice Street, Binghamton, NY 13904-1580
EUROSPAN/Haworth, 3 Henrietta Street, London WC2E 8LU England

Library of Congress Cataloging-in-Publication Data

Fat Oppression and psychotherapy: a feminist perspective / Laura S. Brown, guest editor; Esther D. Rothblum, editor.
   p. cm.
   Published also as Women & Therapy, v. 8, no. 3, 1989. Includes bibliographical references.
   ISBN 0-86656-954-5
   1. Overweight women – Mental health.   2. Obesity – Social aspects.   3. Discrimination against overweight persons.   4. Self – acceptance.   5. Feminist therapy.   I. Brown, Laura S. II. Rothblum, Esther D.
   [DNLM: 1. Discrimination (Psychology)   2. Obesity – psychology.   3. Obesity – therapy. 4. Psychotherapy.   5. Women – psychology.   W1W0433V v. 8 no. 3 / WD 210 F252]
RC552.025F37 1989
616.3'98'0082 – dc20
DNLM/DLC
for Library of Congress   89-19860
                                                              CIP

Fat Oppression and Psychotherapy: A Feminist Perspective

CONTENTS

understanding
obesity

ALL HAWORTH BOOKS & JOURNALS
ARE PRINTED ON CERTIFIED
ACID-FREE PAPER

ABOUT THE EDITORS

Laura S. Brown, PhD, is a clinical psychologist in private practice and Clinical Associate Professor of psychology at the University of Washington in Seattle. Dr. Brown has published a number of papers on the topic of fat oppression in psychotherapy, in addition to her work in the fields of feminist therapy theory, assessment and diagnosis, and ethics. Her paper on feminist therapy with post-traumatic stress disorder won the 1987 Distinguished Publication Award of the Association for Women in Psychology. Dr. Brown is a Diplomate in Clinical Psychology of the American Board of Professional Psychology, and was recently appointed Book Review Editor of the journal *Women & Therapy.*

Esther D. Rothblum, PhD, is Assistant Professor of psychology at the University of Vermont, where she chairs the Women's Studies Program. She is formerly Visiting Scholar at the Institute for Women's Studies, University of Minnesota, Duluth. She is planning a trip to the Antarctic to study gender differences in stress and coping. Currently a Kellogg Fellow, Dr. Rothblum will be traveling to Africa to study women's mental health. In addition, she co-edited the books *The Stereotyping of Women: Its Effects on Mental Health* and *Another Silenced Trauma,* which received a 1987 Distinguished Publication Award from the Association for Women in Psychology. Dr. Rothblum is a co-editor of the journal *Women & Therapy.*

EDITORIAL STATEMENT

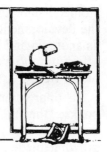

It is with great pleasure that we introduce to our readers this collection of articles on the topic of fat oppression in psychotherapy. We believe that this is a unique work in the professional psychotherapy literature; one that approaches the question of women's experiences with fatness from an anti-fat-oppressive perspective. Although fat activists have been raising the issues that our authors review here for more than a decade, their accumulated wisdom has never been embraced by the practitioners who work with fat women. Therapists, including feminist therapists, have been colluding with their clients in pathologizing fat, celebrating weight loss, and failing to adequately challenge cultural stereotypes of attractiveness for women. In creating this special issue, we hope to take the first step in reversing that trend.

Fat oppression is hatred and discrimination against fat people, primarily fat women, solely because of their body size. It is the stigmatization of being fat, the terror of fat, the rationale for a thousand diets and an equal number of compulsive exercise programs. It is the equation of fat with being out-of-control, with laziness, with deeply-rooted pathology, with ugliness. It is, like physical and sexual violence against women, sexism in action. Internalized fat oppression, which exists in almost all women raised in white North American culture, is a catalyst for energy-draining self-hatred. It leads us to starve ourselves, to life-threatening surgeries such as stomach-stapling and liposuction; it places women at high risk for the development of chronic and intransigent eating disorders such as anorexia and bulimia. It serves to give away our power for self-affirmation to a culture that tells us that we can "never be too thin or too rich," equating value and class status with a starved body.

Fat oppression is also good business. Weight-loss programs, diet books, "health" spas, diet pills; the millions of dollars spent on these, mostly by women, add up. All of this occurs in the face of growing medical evidence that weight is a biologically mediated phenomenon that varies widely throughout the population, and that individual metabolisms vary as widely. A maintenance eating program for one person may consist of over 4,000 daily calories; for another, only 1,200 will suffice. Dieting serves to make the metabolism more efficient, thus ensuring the gaining of weight lost on a diet, and the likelihood of greater gain (Bennett & Gurin, 1982). "Successful" outcomes in research on the long-term effects of very low calorie diets (e.g., less than 600 calories per day) combined with regular aerobic exercise are outcomes where only 80% of the dieters gain back all the weight lost within eighteen months, instead of the usual figures of greater than 90%. Empirical data tell us that all the self-starvation done in the name of health and beauty leads women to feel like failures, while damaging their health in the process.

In this collection of articles, we challenge the notion that fat equals pathology. Additionally, we aim to disconnect the issues of food intake and eating disorders form those of weight. Our perspective is that being fat is simply one variant of human size, not an indication of disordered eating: We have purposely chosen not to include any articles on eating disorders for that reason, so as to create as clear as possible a demarcation between the problems encountered in coping with fat oppression and disordered eating style. Our authors approach fat oppression, not fat, as the problem. They share personal and professional experiences of challenging fat oppression, and offer strategies for therapists to rid themselves of fat oppressive attitudes, as well as intervene in those of clients. They stress the importance of supporting women in learning to love their fat bodies, not as a settling for second best but as a celebration of who they are. These articles challenge cultural myths that have long been taken as truths: that fat is unhealthy, that fat women are physically unfit, that fat women are in hiding from their sexuality or their personal power.

We look forward to feedback from our readers on these articles and hope that they generate further work in this area. We have just begun to integrate anti-fat-oppressive perspectives into the practice of psychotherapy. To do so, we must overcome within ourselves and our colleagues long and firmly held prejudices about the value of being thin. We must deal with our own fears of our female bodies, of being ample, taking space, carrying weight.

Laura S. Brown
Esther D. Rothblum

REFERENCE

Bennett, W., & Gurin, J. (1982) *The dieter's dilemma*. New York: Basic Books.

whoever i am, i'm a fat woman

the space of a silhouette
entering the space of a silence

curvatures of silk
caverns flooding
welcome to a canyon:

she's a horsewoman
a tennis match
a champion runner

she's an artist woman
a desert woman
a dancer

she's a fat woman

a fashion hall for dreams

she's a seeker   your lover   your sister
a dreamer   a bohemian   a thinker
your doctor   she's a healer
a psychic   her stories will set you free

herb lady
masseuse
mathematician
architect
sexologist
clothes designer
museum curator
sculptress
archaeologist

a farmer

a laughter's echo
she's a fat woman
a woman
bound to cut
this earth of the shadows inside her

cliffhanger
ballroom dancer
go-getter
bartender

scene stealer wheeler dealer

a leaper a runner a roller

she's a fat woman and she's breathing

the unknown woman
the woman   who flavours her own song

she's a genius
she's extraordinary
she's an ordinary girl
she's a fat woman

cab driver welder tea drinker
street walker
prude

she's a blues singer
a floutist a drummer

a pin up girl
an ice skater
an icecream lover
a hindu

a hiker a kite flyer
your shadow on the tightrope
she's a fat woman

your shadow
a brake mechanic
a concert cellist

a saxaphonist
leaping on laughter's echo the rhythms of her life.

poet playrite witch nun jew

surfer
bathing beauty
high heeled sexy tramp

scorpio rising
rubenesque pearl

priestess potter shoemaker
hairstylist jeweler
thankyou.   a furniture design.

the woman procurred by money
the woman who is heard above laughter

the woman who walks beyond
the streets of desire
the woman who has always walked these streets
with passion
the woman who has taken over the space of her body
and the woman who has refused to conquer that space.

worker bohemian boss scholar aristocrat
roadrunner sailor weaver

a fat girl
she's a wallflower
socializer leader recluse wanderer

an advertisement for love:
in lillian russell days
you'd follow her
her bare ankles
down the river's muddy edge by foot
making love to her on your knees

she's a stallion   a fleet of rivers.

feel the woman
whose river bathes in mammoth luxury
tracing the moons
that are inside her

she's an aesthetic woman
she's a plastic woman
she's a junkie
a hobo
a housekeeper

candlemaker
chiropractor
stuck up bitch
fast smiler
on welfare or could be
she's a fat woman

the silent woman
worn
with a mask   around herself

the woman who is challenged to a duel

the woman who is tortured

tied to the bed and raped

the woman who always sleeps in black
the woman who never says "excuse me"
or smiles when she's supposed to

the woman who's existence is in question

rough outrageous dull graceful ingenious

exciting to be alive as being a fat woman

she's a deep sea diver
a windmill climber
a motorcycle mama
and a bicycle rider
she's a fat woman

she's a snow shoveler
a short stopper
a wind lover
a heart breaker

certain truths
will make your heart beat fat
when you hear them from a fat woman

you'll grow pale
get chills
disbelieve
but she's marching toward you
she's here and she's taking back her life.

a tough springer
a dead ringer
watch the stones
they throw
her
will turn
to looks of beauty

the stones
they throw to works of art
will turn to looks of beauty.

—Sharonah Robinson

Metamorphosis

Kelly Kay Goodman

SUMMARY. In this article, I indicate that I have spent most of my life in self-hatred, taking abuse from everyone; teachers, peers, family, and society at large. I am a beautiful person, we all are, and I believe that as women it is time we stopped being dictated to by others who rule the diet and fashion industries. It's time that we stopped trying to live up to unrealistic role models. We are individuals who are as different as the colors of the rainbow, and we should be treated as such, and respect each other's differences.

Imagine being denied a snack in kindergarten, and then sent to the hospital for extensive testing simply because you enjoy drinking water and, because you are a fat child, your teacher feels that you may be diabetic. Imagine being "dogpiled" by 22 other children, being singled out as the one who is anti-social, when at every chance you try to be friends with others only to be beaten up or picked on verbally. Think of never having the chance to participate in most school activities, and not being able to defend yourself and your personal possessions against others because no one cares, and when someone does pay attention, it always manages to be seen as your fault. You are not invited to parties, and when you finally get up the courage to apply for a job, you are turned down because other employees feel that, because of your weight, you can't handle the job. Imagine that instead of being fat, you are a woman or a Black, and that these are the only reasons to account for the treat-

Kelly Kay Goodman was born on March 15, 1966, in McCook, NE. She graduated from Wilcox High School, Wilcox, NE, in 1984. She is a member of the United Methodist Church and the International Women's Writing Guild. She is currently pursuing independent research projects on social and political commentary.

11

ment by others. We call this prejudice, and consider this unfair and shameful behavior. Yet the person who experienced these injustices wasn't Black; the person was a fat child, teenager, and is now a fat woman. Should this type of prejudice be taken any less seriously? The answer should be, but has rarely been no.

I am not weak-willed; I have tried diet after diet to no avail. I have spent most of my life in self-hatred, taking abuse from everyone; teachers, peers, family, and society at large. I am a beautiful person, we all are, and I believe that as women it is time we stopped being dictated to by others who rule the diet and fashion industries. It's time that we stopped trying to live up to unrealistic role models. We are individuals who are as different as the colors of the rainbow, and we should be treated as such.

We must stop this endless cycle of self-abuse; we must finally realize that all we hear from the doctors, media, diet and fashion industries, are based upon making money. Did you ever stop to consider that if all those so-called weight-loss saints care so much for fat people, why don't they offer their weight-loss services at no charge? After all, if our health is truly what they're concerned with, why don't they offer their services free? What about fat people who can't afford these services? We must once and for all see that the "we-can-be-anything-for-the-right-amount-of-money" is nothing more than snake oil salesmanship. We are being told that we must be slim to be healthy, but we have to realize that this is not true. Medical facts have long been both suppressed and manipulated by the AMA to support the theory that being fat is being "at risk" and unhealthy. Being fat is a physical characteristic, not a disease.

Imagine if scientists developed a pill to turn Blacks into Whites and told you, a Black, through every type of media and through every doctor over and over again that in order to be a worthwhile person you *must* be White. If you took those pills (and you know you would because they have convinced you that you're a bad, unworthy, unhuman person), and if those pills didn't work for you, and it wasn't because you didn't want them to work or didn't follow the instructions exactly, and the media and medical professions continued to tell you that you will die unless you turned White and that no one will love you. You will never find a job; you are labeled weak-willed, and as a person you are a failure. Wouldn't you start to believe it all after a while? Now suppose all this took place because no matter how much you tried, or no matter how many pills you took, you couldn't become White; and although it's been proven that being Black is a genetic trait, they still tell you and everyone around you that you *could* be White if you really wanted to be.

So the peer pressure is incredible, and because of all this pressure you develop high-blood pressure and related signs of stress, and you know what your doctor says caused it; the fact that you couldn't become White. Neither that doctor, nor the rest of society for that matter, will ever admit that the stress of trying to turn White is the reason for the high-blood pressure or related ailments. They all point the finger at you for "failing" to become White. And society will react towards you to reinforce those feelings of guilt and failure; it will always be your fault that you're still Black.

If you think that this is silly, it isn't. This is happening to people who are fat. We can no more be expected to change the fact that we're fat than to be expected to change the color of our skin. Granted, there are people who overeat, but it is now a proven fact in study after study that most fat people eat no more than their thin counterparts, and in some cases, it has been proven that they actually consume less. People who are fat from birth will always be fat. We have more fat cells than thin people, and less than 2% of all people who diet to lose weight succeed in permanent weight-loss. Diets fail at taking and keeping the weight off, but succeed at making us feel like worthless, weak-willed failures. Yet, we accept the pablum that is spoon-fed to us by the media megabuck diet and fashion industries, without realizing that they're *only* in business to make money. As long as we keep believing their lies, they keep making money in the billions yearly at the expense of our self-worth, self-love, and self-acceptance. They know we will believe anything if they put enough money into advertising; they know that we will continue to be led like lambs to the slaughter house until all of our free will is gone, not to mention our money.

All of my life, since I can remember, I have been picked on about my weight. Since the first day I attended school to the last, I not only had to battle the physical (from classmates), but mental/emotional abuse from peers, teachers, and family, not to mention society at large. I was always told that "children are just that way," suggesting that their verbal and physical abuse was somehow normal and acceptable. But there is never an excuse for cruelty. Never were my feelings taken seriously; I was told by my family and teachers that if I would lose weight they wouldn't treat me that way. Because of this abuse I became very depressed. At age twelve, my mother took me to a psychologist who proceeded to tell me that the reason that none of the diets I had been on since age 5 worked was because I was afraid of boys! I wasn't, but this statement gave my mother more ammunition for the unrelenting pressure to diet. When I was younger, I thought that she was right, and I too believed that I must lose weight to fit in. But luckily, through my early encounters with boys who liked big girls, I learned that what I had always been told, which was, in order to have a boyfriend or be loved, you had to be thin, was untrue. At age 13, while volunteering at a school for the mentally retarded, I met a boy who also was working there who was sixteen; we had a wonderful time together and before long he was my boyfriend. However, the lady who ran the center tried to discredit the relationship with the remark: "See . . . if you can have a boy like you at this size (260 lbs.) imagine how many boys will like you when you are thin." No matter where I turned, I was met at every corner with diets and people telling me that I must be thin. I dreaded going to the doctor, who blamed everything, even a common cold, on my weight.

If you think that I am still fat from lack of trying to lose weight, you are both right and wrong. Before I stopped dieting, I had a history of constant dieting which began at age 5 on "doctor's orders" (I weighed 90 lbs. at that age). I continued to diet and tried every kind of diet and weight-loss system ever devised. Here is a partial list of the "diet products and services" that I have tried: Weight Watchers, NutriSystem, Diet Center, Weight Loss Clinic, The Physician's Diets, The Liquid Protein Diet, Ayds Candy Plan, Dexatrim Plan, Accutrim, Cambridge, Herbalife, Shakelee, Sego, Carnation Diet Bars and Mix, Slim Fast, Richard Simmons, Women Doctor's Diet, Scarsdale Diet, Pritikin Program, The Stillman Diet, The Beverly Hills Diet, The Meat and Potatoes Diet—all types of clinics, books, powders, and devices; in short, any means to lose weight.

At age 12, I attended a weight-loss camp for eight weeks, where they tried to tear down my self-esteem even more. The weight-loss was minimal, and was soon regained. I continued to diet off and on for several years after that. During my junior year in high school, I found a magazine, and I began to feel that my feelings and impressions about the diet game were correct. I started treating myself better; stopped dieting, bought myself clothes that fit, and took care of myself. It all paid off when a boy that I liked in my class asked me out on a date during the junior class play, of which I was student director. I could see that the dieting game wasn't the answer.

I noticed that people around me who were thin, or dieting to be thin, weren't any happier than I was. When I was a child, I couldn't understand this because they were thin, and we all know that thin people are happy, right? Now I know better.

All fat women have been taught for so long that all of our unhappiness and disappointments will be solved if we lose weight and become thin. But I know that this is wrong; we are all individuals and we deserve to be treated as such. Whenever we hear of people who have lost weight and now have more friends, and whose lives seem better, does it never occur to us that this person, because they lost weight, gains social support in all corners of their life? Therefore, they feel better about themselves, so their self-esteem rises artificially; it's as if they were taking a drug to induce a euphoric state, making them feel better and giving them the confidence to pursue things that they wouldn't have when they were fat. Of course, there are people who lose weight and maintain their weight-loss and happiness, but what about those whose happiness is directly linked to their weight-loss with all of its peer and social approval? What happens to these people when the applause stops for their weight-loss? I would guess that they go back to feeling as before, depressed, with low self-esteem, because all that they changed was their outward appearance and they failed to change the inner feelings. So what have they really gained? A few moments of acceptance and a continued life of low self-esteem and new hurt and confusion at the lack of good feelings they have for themselves. Now they fit the outward appearance of a happy, healthy person, while inwardly they remain the same. People accept you when you lose weight because society has been taught that you are in control and a worthwhile person if you are thin. But when you are fat, you are not considered to be in control nor to be a worthwhile person. This isn't a truth, but a media-fabricated lie.

Self-esteem is one of the hardest things for us as humans to develop. From the time we are born, we are judged, labeled, and herded into groups; we face, for the most part, a life designed for us by others. If we are ever lucky enough to realize this sad fact, it is almost always too late for us to change, so we believe. We make it so hard for ourselves to find self-acceptance and love; we live all of our lives to make money, raise families, build security, and most of all to strive for social acceptance.

We need to take care of ourselves now. We need to stop worrying about what others will think; so much of the time we confirm people's attitudes and beliefs about us by the way we act. If we act unhappy, uncomfortable, or all-out miserable, people will take the only information that they have, our body language and their own misconceptions, and they will assume that we are unhappy because we are fat. This only reinforces their misguided attitudes and beliefs.

Rebuilding one's self-esteem after years of having it torn down is never an easy process, and it certainly isn't fast. I started rebuilding my own self-esteem when, by chance, I came across that magazine for big women when I was seventeen. I can't tell you how to rebuild your own self-esteem, but, here are a few things that helped me: (1) I started reading everything that I could about fat acceptance, (2) I joined organizations and subscribed to magazines and friendship correspondence clubs that supported the fat-is-beautiful ideal, (3) I attended as many social functions as possible which cater to larger-size people and their admirers, (4) I examined how society is brainwashed and manipulated by the media and medical establishments, along with the fashion and diet industries, (5) I searched for clothes that fit me and slowly but surely built a wardrobe of new clothing that not only fit, but that I felt comfortable in, (6) I took care of myself and did things for me that I had deprived myself of for so long, such as getting a facial makeover, a manicure, and just getting out and enjoying life. But the thing that helped me the most was realizing that I wasn't alone and that others felt beautiful being fat too. Slowly but surely, over a period of years, I rebuilt my self-esteem.

Stop sometime when you are out in public and just people-watch. You will find that people come in all shapes and sizes and colors, and they all have something about them that makes them truly individual and special. Most importantly, I stopped dieting, and my body found its own setpoint of weight and metabolism. No matter how much or how little I eat, my weight stays within a few pounds of my setpoint. The hardest thing to do is to dare to be yourself. When people learn that they can't get a rise out of you when they make rude comments about your weight, eventually they will stop. And those who do not; well, after a while you don't hear them, and if you do, they don't matter anyway! What if your friends and family don't accept you? If they don't, they were never your friends to begin with. Friends stick by you because of who *you* are, *not* because you fit their aesthetic criteria. As far as family, mine won't accept me and I figure that's their loss. I'm a wonderfully beautiful, intelligent woman, and if they don't want to be around me because I am fat, that's okay! After all, who needs people who are so shallow as to allow their feelings about someone they love to be influenced by the "mighty media money machine" Through the clubs that I have joined, I met many people who have similar viewpoints about weight as I do. I even met my husband through a personal ad. He has always found fat women beautiful. He is no different than a man who finds thin women attractive; he is being honest with his feelings, and he is a happy, successful, attractive, loving man whom I wouldn't trade for anything nor anyone. Most of all, I feel happy and finally at peace with myself, no more torture nor self-hatred; it's unnecessary because fat is beautiful! It is a state of mind of inner peace and self-acceptance, and I only wish that all women could find the happiness that I have found, because I can't imagine life being any better than this. Remember, don't let anyone, especially yourself, tell you that you can't do something; you can do anything if you set your mind to it. But the first step is self-love. Because with self-love comes peace, and when you are finally at peace, the world is a place of opportunity, not a place that you wish to escape from. Life is a wonderful experience, if only you allow yourself to live it and enjoy it fully!

Until the women of this world accept each other, regardless of race, ethnic background, religion, and especially size, we can never sincerely hope to be taken seriously by others.

If we continue to believe that supposed "cures" to what allegedly "ails" us can be had in a jar or in a clinic for a small fortune, we can never hope to move forward. We as sisters must no longer accept the chains of self-hatred that bind us. We must overcome this system and the negative feelings that it causes, and truly realize that we are all special and that there is a place in this world for all of us, not just the ones who fit the ideal of an economic system. We must realize that we can be both feminine AND strong, and that the one all-powerful way for us to show our strength is through our handling of the dollar. Stop buying products in hopes of becoming a woman that society is dictating you must become. Dare to be who you are; a beautiful, powerful, intelligent woman who is truly an individual, who can do anything that she sets her mind to. Not a woman coerced into self-doubt and self-hatred by a media dollar-induced social attitude. We can refuse to allow the system make us dislike ourselves. Know that we are individuals and that our inner strength is strong enough to be the women we are, not the women that they want us to be. Let social change start with us. Let the buck stop here/today with us. Remember without financial support, these morbid money machines can't continue. We must stop shelling out the money to perpetuate their system. Instead of buying those diet aids, that we don't really need, let's have a manicure, buy a pair of shoes, or a good dinner, but in all cases, pamper ourselves. I guarantee that we'll feel better and that our self-esteems will thank us.

One last word, I should tell you that I am 5'2" tall and over 500 lbs., and 22 years of age. I have been happily married for over four years, and I love myself. Life is a pleasure for me; make it a pleasure for yourself!

Tell them that you won't take it anymore by getting out there and flexing your financial muscle. *Dare to be yourself!!*

Fat-Oppressive Attitudes and the Feminist Therapist: Directions for Change

Laura S. Brown

SUMMARY. This article will examine the responses of other feminist therapists to the author's anti-fat-oppressive stance. These reactions will be used as a base from which to generate some hypotheses regarding the difficulties that continue to be faced by women therapists in attempts to identity and reduce internalized fat-oppressive attitudes regarding their own bodies and those of their women clients. Suggestions for heightening personal awareness regarding internalized fat oppression, and strategies for reducing fat-oppressive attitudes as a therapist will be presented.

I. INTRODUCTION

This article will address one of feminist therapy's "problems that have no name"; the continuing presence of overt and covert fat-oppressive attitudes among feminist therapists. Fat oppression, which can be defined as the fear and hatred of fat people, particularly women, and the concomitant presence of oppressive and discriminatory practices aimed toward fat people, has become one of the few "acceptable" prejudices still held by otherwise progressive

Laura S. Brown, PhD, is a feminist therapist in private practice and Clinical Associate Professor of Psychology at the University of Washington in Seattle. She is the author of numerous articles and book chapters on topics in feminist therapy, with special interest in women and fat oppression, lesbian issues, feminist therapy theory, ethics, and assessment and diagnosis. She is active nationally in psychological organizations as a voice for feminist therapy and lesbian and gay issues, and is a Diplomate in Clinical Psychology of the American Board of Professional Psychology.

19

and aware persons (Scoenfielder & Weiser, 1983). Fat oppression is particularly aimed at women, and has been analyzed by a number of authors as being one of the various ways in which patriarchal oppression is insinuated into women's lives, having impact in a profound and persistent way on the most intimate aspects of our lives. As I have commented in earlier writings, fat oppression leads women to fear feeding and nourishing themselves, thus depriving ourselves of both strength and pleasure (Brown, 1985, 1987). Fat oppression carries the less-than-subtle message that women are forbidden to take up space (by being large of body) or resources (by eating food ad libitum). Fat oppression also serves to divide women and drain energy and resources from women's lives. The weight-loss industry, which preys upon the fear of fat fostered by fat-oppressive attitudes, robs women of millions of dollars yearly which could be spent in other, non-self-destructive manners. This industry, and fat oppression in general, encourage competition between women to be "the thinnest of them all," a race which has had deadly outcomes in the rising rates of eating disorders such as anorexia nervosa and bulimia, which have at their core the terror of becoming fat.

The fact that fat-oppressive attitudes exist among feminist therapists is in many ways not strange given that most of those who identify themselves as feminist therapists are women, a group in which internalized fat-oppressive attitudes are powerfully present. This is not to suggest that any group of therapists is free from fat-oppressive values; certainly male therapists and non-feminist women therapists have long histories of acting in biased and fat-oppressive manners towards their women clients of all body sizes. Rather, it is more surprising to encounter such an entrenched oppressive attitude among a group of therapists who are committed to a political analysis of the work of psychotherapy. However, data suggests that North American women of most cultures, and all body size and eating styles tend to have fat-oppressive and fat-negative attitudes towards their own bodies and, by inference, those of other women (Rodin, Silberman & Striegel-Moore, 1985). Such attitudes towards fat and especially, fat women, are, unlike other oppressive perspectives such as racism, sexism, homophobia, and ageism which feminist therapist have actively sought out in themselves and rejected, often embraced, excused or rationalized by therapists on the grounds that fat per se is unhealthy, that its presence is *prima facie* evidence of unexpressed intrapsychic conflicts and that it is thus a target worthy of stigma and intervention. Even among feminist therapists with our supposedly heightened awareness of the danger to women present in cultural demands for female thinness, fat oppression, usually subtly expressed, is still the norm.

This paper will explore and review the themes I have found in female and feminist therapist colleagues' responses to my work as a writer of anti-fat-oppressive feminist therapy theory. I will use these responses as a source of data regarding the attitudes of therapists towards fat, their own and that of other women, and as a stepping-off point from which to explore the problem of continued fat oppression in the practice of feminist therpay. I will suggest strategies for heightened self-awareness in therapists regarding their own internalized fat oppression and its impact on their work. My operating hypothesis is that fat-oppressive attitudes (e.g., the stigmatizing of fatness and the glorification and active promulgation of thinness) are themselves a variant of sexism and misogyny (see Chernin, 1981 for a more complete exegesis of this concept), and that their continued presence in the therapy context is indicative of an ethically questionable stance by the therapist, particularly in those therapists with a commitment to non-sexist perspectives in their work.

II. ENCOUNTERING FAT OPPRESSION AMONG COLLEAGUES

In the early 1980s I began to write and speak about the concept of fat oppression in psychotherapy, and to present an anti-fat-oppressive feminist theoretical analysis of the social constructs of weight and eating (Brown, 1983a, 1983b, 1985, 1986, 1987). Much of what I was developing in this series of papers came from three sources: my own previous experiences as a (formerly) fat girl and woman; the clinical materials regarding attitudes towards food, weight, eating, and dieting presented by *all* of my women clients, irrespective of size; and feminist writings against fat oppression (Schoenfielder & Wieser, 1983), most of which had been created by fat women themselves. Retrospectively, I can see the remnants of my own internalized fat-oppressive attitudes in my choice of timing. I only began to do this work in public after my body had reversed course and without conscious effort became significantly smaller. Thus, I had unconsciously required myself to obtain the privileges of a woman who can buy her clothes off the rack in any store (a good operational definition of a non-fat woman; while I am still considered "overweight" by the insurance company charts, those illogical sources of so-called truth on what sizes we should all be, I am no longer fat) before I would allow myself to speak publicly and with authority on this topic.

Also in retrospect, I can see why this may have unfortunately been the wisest choice. I say "unfortunately" because of the types of responses I have encountered among many of my colleagues. I am nearly certain that, were I still clearly a fat woman I would have encountered even more discounting and fat-oppressive responses to my work than I actually have. Worse, I probably would never had heard it outright; fat oppression, while pervasive, is generally considered impolite when overtly expressed to a fat person. (Covert expressions are, however, considered extremely positive; more than once I was "complimented" by people on my own weight loss and "attractiveness," including during periods of time when I was so obviously ill or exhausted that no one could have found my appearance appealing. And we are all familiar with "She has such a pretty face," the damning-with-faint-praise aimed at fat women.) Only once did an anonymous reviewer of a paper, safely hidden behind her identifying letter, state in so many words that which I had inferred from the carefully worded questions of others. She wrote that the only reason that I could possibly be espousing these attitudes was because I was some sort of fat activist (read "biased fat person") attempting to sneak my strange ideas through the back door disguised as feminist therapy theory.

This reviewer's comments reflect what I believe to be one of the common themes in the reactions of women therapists toward my work: extreme discomfort with the notion that being fat is not the problem, but being fat-oppressed and/or fat-oppressive is. The beliefs that fat is dangerous, disfiguring, unhealthy, the result of disordered eating, indicative of a fear of sex/femininity/success (pick your favorite and fill in the blank), and to be avoided at almost all

costs have the flavor of religious faith. They are embraced and prac-
ticed by so many women, including female and feminist therapists,
that to suggest otherwise can bring charges of heresy.

This "true-believer" type of response often took the form of pre-
senting me with clinical case examples of "my obese client whose
doctor said she would die if she didn't lose weight," (these being
among the few instances in which feminist therapists of my ac-
quaintance appeared willing to take on faith the pronouncements of
male physicians regarding the health needs of their clients) or stories of clients whose "successful" weight loss had *truly* helped
their self-esteem (chillingly analogous to pre-feminist literature on
women who had learned to "accept their femininity" and become
happier as a result).

I would attempt to parry these supposedly prohibitive examples
of "fat-is-the-problem" with the hefty literature on the health risks
of dieting (a literature that is almost entirely ignored by the medica-
lized weight-loss establishment), particularly the repetitive dieting
patterns that are so typical of North American women, or would try
to remind my readers/listeners that most fat people are healthy and
at less risk from their size than from the negative and prejudicial
attitudes of others. This was usually to no avail; although the literature on weight and body size increasingly supports an anti-fat-oppressive perspective (for instance demonstrating that body size is
more likely to be a function of heredity than of modifiable eating
styles, and that fat people can be and often are as fit and healthy as
non-fat people, with true health risks only lying at both the extreme
low and extreme high ends of the weight continuum), the belief
system which supports fat oppression is a powerful one indeed. No
matter how much data I gathered to bolster my arguments, I found
them falling on closed ears more often than not.

A second frequent response to my work was the implication that I
wouldn't feel this way if I weren't/hadn't been fat myself. The less
than subtle message was that to be anti-fat-oppressive was a defen-
sive stance that I was taking in order to rationalize my own "unac-
ceptable" past status. I was "colluding" with my fat clients to keep
fat so that I could feel okay about not being thin myself.

Such a charge of non-conscious bias would be funnier if it
weren't the case that most of my "friendly, caring" interlocutors

were themselves demonstrating bias, one so pervasive as to be invisible to them. A parallel can easily be drawn to equally spurious concerns that lesbian or gay therapists who are comfortable and positive with their own sexuality would be biased toward homosexuality in such a way as to make them insufficiently objective in working with people who were exploring sexual identity. The heterosexist bias held by most therapists is rarely considered in this argument because of the non-conscious assumption that to be pro-heterosexuality is *not* a bias but rather an expression of the "truth." So, similarly being anti-fat is perceived by most North Americans as simply the right and only way to be, with pro-fat and anti-fat-oppressive perspectives singled out as a peculiar and deviant bias to be guarded against.

My sense is, additionally, that challenging one's own internalized fat oppression is a uniquely difficult and painful task for most women therapist, particularly those who have never been fat but who have "felt fat" and dieted for much of their adult lives, a state common to many women. When I suggest that my colleagues begin to develop anti-fat-oppressive attitudes in their work, I am asking them to call into question personal issues that may have been organizing principles of their lives. What I am saying, in essence, is that their diets have had no meaning, that their repetitive struggles to be "just ten pounds thinner" are probably futile, that the two-sizes-smaller piece of clothing that has hung in the closet as the symbol of success and attractiveness might just as well be donated to the battered women's shelter clothing bank. I am asking them to feel "out-of-control," the term most often used by women to describe the experience of not watching their weight (Roth, 1982, 1984). I am telling them that all their work with clients to help the latter lose weight have been oppressive and are likely to generate further difficulties for those clients somewhere in their lives; I am pointing out to feminist therapists how they have colluded with sexism and the hatred of women. I am asking my female colleagues to challenge the foundations upon which their sense of personal attractiveness and desirability has been built. Although such confrontations are delivered in what I hope is a tactful and educative manner, I realize that it is easier for many of my colleagues to respond defensively than it is to begin the very risky yet necessary personal work of examining their own internalized fat oppression. I can only guess that what I encounter is an echo of what women of color must hear each time they remind white women such as myself of our omnipresent racism.

A final theme of these responses is guilt. Many feminist therapists, when exposed to the concept of fat oppression, will quickly recognize it within themselves and resolve to change, yet still feel bound to its dictates. There is likely to be enormous cognitive dissonance; feminist principles of non-oppressiveness will battle with North American female socialization which, although emanating from white culture, has impact on women of all colors and cultures in North America, to desire and value thinness. This struggle may be further complicated for women who are in other ways distant from the white, blond ideal of female beauty, for whom thinness is one of few apparent avenues of access to a marginally "acceptable" self-presentation.

Such women will speak furtively of envying their bulimic women clients who can "eat as much as they want and get away with it," not yet realizing how such statements reflect the fat-oppressive worship of thinness while totally discounting the pain and inordinate health risks of bulimia. They will admit to their own fears of being fat, yet experience themselves as helpless to modify those feelings because of the social and personal contingencies operating in their lives: "how can I feel secure in my own relationship if I gain weight?" (begging the question of how they can sustain themselves, or support any woman, in remaining in relationships in which they are abused because of their size. One interesting note here; some recent research has shown that internalized fat-oppressive attitudes are more present in persons of *either* gender who want to be found attractive by men, while they occur at lower rates in persons of either gender who wish to be found attractive by women [Siever, 1988]. These data strongly underline the connection between sexism and fat oppression). These therapists will feel guilty for being fat-oppressive, but believe that there is no choice but to maintain those beliefs in some way.

Such guilt functions as an obstacle to careful and reflective self-examination and may temporarily serve to increase covert fat-oppressive attitudes while generating superficial external behavioral movement in the direction of being more fat-affirmative. This can lead to the expression of confusing double messages both to self and to clients; one therapist, for instance, told her clients that it was okay to be fat, but ostentatiously participated in a modified liquid fasting diet program. The message was that while it was acceptable for *clients* to be fat women, *therapists*, as so-called models of good functioning, were required to stay thin. Most therapists who are mired in feelings of guilt or shame about their fat-oppressive attitudes are likely to engage in similar, although less strikingly obvious behaviors while they are attempting to move through their feelings to a more satisfactory, clearly thought-through resolution. Guilt creates difficulty in thinking clearly, and slows this process.

III. CORRECTIVE MEASURES

A first step towards an anti-fat-oppressive stance is the acknowledgement of one's own fat-oppressive attitudes. There need be no shame in this. Just as white North American women learn to be sexist, racist, and homophobic, almost all North American women also learn to hate and fear fatness, particularly in ourselves. I have suggested that a fat woman by her presence violates primal norms of misogynist society that deny nurturance, space, power, and visibility to women (Brown, 1985, 1987) in the way that lesbians violate the norm that women must be dependent of and deferent to men. Becoming more fat-oppressive is often an indicator of assimilation and acculturation; the immigrant woman who valued fat in her children as a symbol of being well-fed and healthy is often the grandmother of the bulimic woman who hates and fears her genetically generated "zoftig" breasts and thighs. The stereotype of the poor, fat welfare mother is contrasted with the images of thin, successful women entrepreneurs. We can acknowledge the power of a non-conscious ideology (Bem & Bem, 1976) without blaming ourselves, its victims and survivors, for having internalized it unknowing.

A second step is self-awareness and self-exploration to determine how fat oppression expresses itself in our own lives. This is a sort of a "coming-out" process, a reevaluation and embrace of that which has previously been stigmatized and made ego-alien within ourselves, our fat and all which surrounds it cognitively and affectively. I would like to suggest that while first engaging in this process of personal consciousness raising it is probably unwise and possibly unethical to work with women who are dealing directly with issues of food, weight, eating, or body image. Gonsiorek (1987), addressing a parallel issue, has suggested that lesbian and gay therapists in the process of coming out not work with lesbian and gay clients until they are themselves settled and certain with their own sexual orientation and identity. He points out that during the early stages of coming out, when there is likely to be much ambivalence and continued expression of internalized homophobia, lesbian and gay therapists are at some risk to act oppressively and potentially unethically with their sexual minority clients as a form of acting out of that ambivalence and self-hatred, yet may seek out such clients as part of their attempts at self-affirmation. Similarly, a woman therapist beginning to struggle with her own internalized fat oppression may wish to fill her practice with fat clients as a way of externally manifesting her new, "converted" status at a point when she may still be many steps behind those clients in coping with the impact of societal fat oppression on a variety of aspects of functioning.

It is, rather, essential to acknowledge how powerful and pervasive are fat-oppressive attitudes and actions in the lives of women, including female therapists, and to create the kind of non-fat-oppressive social support and professional consultation which would tend to facilitate well-integrated attitude changes. If we work with or refer to physicians or other primary health care providers we need to ascertain their attitudes towards an anti-fat-oppressive stance, and allow ourselves to support our clients' rights *not* to go on diets or be weighed at medical appointments.

Self-help is also an option. This includes attending to how often we engage in fat-oppressive self-statements, e.g., saying, "I feel fat," when what we mean is "I feel bad," or making comments about how much exercise we will have to do to "work off" the food we are now eating. Additionally, we must carefully examine our feelings about those of our clients who may resemble the cultural ideals of thinness more closely than we do. Do we envy them their looks or discount their distress because they are "thin and pretty"?

Such exploration can also extend itself to our attitudes towards the body sizes of our women friends and family members. Particularly if we are the struggling to be thin daughters of a fat mother (fathers, being men apparently are less threatening in their fat, both because it tends to be less forbidden to men and because of the gender barrier which decreases our tendency to identify with the male parent) we may find ourselves acting out our fat oppression with shame at being seen in the presence of our fat relatives and the desire to dissociate ourselves from fat women, whoever they may be, out of the primitive fear that fat will be contagious.

We can also attend to language. The term "overweight" implies an excess above an ideal weight; it is used incorrectly as interchangeable with "fat," which is erroneous. "Fat" is a descriptive term which, stripped of its cultural baggage, has no necessary implications of wrongness or deviation (imagine for a minute the parallel terms: "undermale" as the equivalent of "female," for instance). "Obese" similarly implies a medicalization of a bodily size, with the meta-message of pathology. We also need to check our assumptions about how eating and weight are and are not related. Disordered eating comes with all body sizes and types, as does self-regulated, comfortable eating. We need to be attentive to the possibility that we only suggest eating chocolate or buying new clothes as self-nurturing devices to our thin clients; again, are we subtly saying that only the small of body deserve nourishment?

Finally, and as with all forms of internalized oppression as factors in the therapy process, we can empower our clients with knowledge and with the expressed right to confront us when our undetected fat-oppressive attitudes surface in therapy. For instance, my waiting room contains copies of *Radiance*, the anti-fat-oppressive magazine by and for fat women. Reading it introduces many of my clients for the first time to the notion that fat is simply another size, and also a culturally oppressed group, opening the door for discussion of fat oppression during therapy, and enlightening my clients about their options when I stumble over my own unacknowledged internalized fat oppressiveness. I also attempt to keep current with research on body size and its various sources, and to make that information available to clients who are struggling with their own feelings of being too big and thus the wrong size. In this instance, it is extraordinarily helpful that the available empirical literature so strongly supports an anti-fat-oppressive stance, since the popular and self-help literature are among the worst offenders as sources of fat-oppressive constructs.

Fat oppression has no place in psychotherapy; it is, however, a powerful cultural current that is difficult for many women unambivalently to challenge. By becoming aware of the many and subtle ways in which our internalized fat oppression as women enters our lives and attitudes, we are less likely to either pass the oppression along to clients, or encourage and collude with it when it comes from within them.

REFERENCES

Bem, S. & Bem, D. (1976) Training the woman to know her place: The power of a non-conscious ideology. In S. Cox (Ed.) *Female psychology: The emerging self*. Chicago: SRA, Inc.

Brown, L.S. (1983a, March) *"Overweight" and "overeating"; The standards and their impact on women*. Paper presented at the Conference of the Association for Women in Psychology, Seattle WA.

Brown, L.S. (1983b, May) *Women, weight, and power*. Paper presented at the Second Advanced Feminist Therapy Institute, Washington DC.

Brown, L.S. (1985) Women, weight and power: Feminist theoretical and therapeutic issues. *Women & Therapy*, *4*, pp. 61-71.

Brown, L.S. (1986, August) Fat oppression and psychotherapy: A new look at the meaning of body size. In K. Brehony (Chair) *Women in context: Disordered or displaced*. Symposium presented at the Convention of the American Psychological Association, Washington DC.

Brown, L.S. (1987) Lesbians, weight and eating: New analysis and perspectives. In Boston Lesbian Psychologies Collective (Eds.) *Lesbian Psychologies* (pp. 294-309). Urbana/Chicago: University of Illinois Press.

Chernin, K. (1981) *The obsession: Reflections on the tyranny of slenderness*. New York: Harper/Colophon.

Gonsiorek, J. (1987, August) Ethical issues for lesbian and gay psychotherapists. In L. Garnets (Chair) *Developing conceptual frameworks for ethical decision-making*. Symposium presented at the Convention of the American Psychological Association, New York NY.

Rodin, J., Silberman, L., & Streigel-Moore, R. (1985) Women and weight: A normative discontent. In T. Sonderegger (Ed.) *Psychology and gender*. Lincoln NE: University of Nebraska Press.

Roth, G. (1982) *Feeding the hungry heart: The experience of compulsive eating*. New York: New American Library.

Roth, G. (1984) *Breaking free from compulsive eating*. Indianapolis: Bobbs-Merrill.

Schoenfielder, L. & Weiser, B. (Eds.) (1983) *Shadow on a tightrope: Writings by women on fat oppression*. Iowa City: Aunt Lute Book Company.

Siever, M. (1988, August) *Sexual orientation, gender, and the perils of sexual objectification*. Paper presented at the Convention of the American Psychological Association, Atlanta GA.

Should Feminist Therapists Do Weight Loss Counseling?

Joan C. Chrisler

SUMMARY. This article presents arguments for and against weight loss counseling in feminist therapy. Conflicts between feminist therapy and weight loss counseling are explored and the implications of counseling and not counseling on women's empowerment are considered. Although each case requires an individual ethical decision, the author, a feminist therapist who has done weight loss counseling in the past, concludes that the answer to the title question should, in general, be "no."

For several years I worked as a therapist leading weight loss groups. The groups were based in hospitals and targeted at people with medical problems; many of my clients were diabetic, hypertensive, arthritic, or recovering from heart attacks. This was an exciting time in my professional development. I learned a great deal about group dynamics, the application of cognitive and behavioral techniques, nutrition and exercise, and the physiology of eating and weight.

However, I always felt conflicted and somewhat guilty about my work. Ever conscious of feminist theory, I discouraged my clients from choosing specific target weights and concentrated on the importance of feeling healthy and finding a weight at which they felt comfortable. No low calorie diets were recommended; the program's emphasis was on learning healthy behavior and making food choices that were right for the participants as individuals. We talked often in the groups about not expecting one's personality to change

Joan C. Chrisler is an experimental psychologist and Assistant Professor of Psychology at Connecticut College. She received postgraduate training in cognitive behavior therapy.

as a result of weight loss and not waiting for weight loss to do things
one really wanted to do. I stressed the importance of self-acceptance at every stage. Yet, each week the clients were weighed and I
found myself congratulating those who had lost weight and consoling those who had gained or remained the same. In doing this I was
surely overriding the feminist messages I had delivered earlier.

Of course, not all my clients had medical conditions. Many
healthy fat women, and some who were well within the average
weight range, managed to get the physician's signature that was
necessary to join a group. I constantly struggled with the desire to
tell these women to save their money and go home! I knew that
encouraging them to lose weight was only playing into their inse-
curities, self-doubts, and concerns about their appearance. I won-
dered whether it is ever feminist to do weight loss counseling as
behavioral medicine. Or should we avoid any activities that reinforce cultural stereotypes regardless of our motives?

BACKGROUND

Central to feminist therapy is the belief that oppressive social
structures have limited women's experiences and shaped women's
status (Ballou & Gabalac, 1985). Obvious among these social structures is the cultural expectation that women will be beautiful and the
cultural current demand in the U.S. for white women is that to be
beautiful one must be thin.

The lengths to which women will go to meet these cultural standards paint a distressing picture. Eichenbaum and Orbach (1983)
estimate that two percent of adolescent girls are anorexic, up to
50% of college women are bulimic, and 60% of adult women are
compulsive eaters who feel constant guilt. In fact, obsessions with
weight and eating have become so common among women in the
U.S. that they now constitute the norm (Rodin, Silberstein &
Striegel-Moore, 1985).

Cultural expectations for beauty have been joined in recent years
by cultural insistence on the pursuit of health. Health food stores,
running shoes, and vitamins have become as popular as diet books
and exercise salons, and, of course, we are told that thin is healthy.
While no one would argue against striving to maintain health (Su-

san B. Anthony insisted that women will need both intellectual and physical strength to win equal rights), it has become an obsession for many people and has taken on moral overtones. This has provided yet another reason for thin women and compulsive exercisers to reject those who don't share their goals (Freedman, 1986).

Medical studies have suggested that weight is correlated with such disorders as diabetes and hypertension, and physicians regularly refer their patients to therapists for weight loss counseling. Yet, it is unclear at what weight such risks for medical illness actually increase (Keys, 1980). One rarely hears about the fact that weight does have medical advantages; increased fat storage means one is more likely to survive a famine and that one has a better prognosis for recovery from tuberculosis and cancer (Fitzgerald, 1981). Many techniques for weight loss (e.g., liquid protein, amphetamines, stomach stapling, jaw wiring, gastric balloons) are more dangerous than maintaining the weight.

THE CASE FOR WEIGHT LOSS COUNSELING

One can argue that weight loss for medical reasons does not conflict with feminist theory. The medical establishment has long promoted the opinion that weight loss may reduce the need for hypertensive medication and can, in some cases, reduce the need for insulin injections in diabetics (Editorial, 1987).[1] After weight loss, one may feel more comfortable physically thus making it easier to increase one's activity level, which helps arthritis and heart disease. Of course, these examples refer to significant weight loss in very fat people, not to the loss of a few pounds by persons within or near the average weight range.

Effective counseling can prevent women from damaging themselves through dangerous weight loss techniques, and from the waste of effort and loss of self-esteem that result from diets and other strategies that don't work. The feminist therapist has the opportunity to disabuse her clients of the myths of willpower and the morality of thinness, and emphasize the inevitability of set-backs. Clear descriptions of the physiology of weight loss/gain relieve guilt and explain why some individuals will never be thin regardless of their behavior.

Feminist therapists have the opportunity to explain why diets don't work. They can discuss with their clients how to make food choices, which includes giving oneself permission to eat high calorie favorites in moderation without guilt. In this way we can work against the "normative" food obsessions while we help our clients to feel comfortable with their weight, rather than a low, perhaps more culturally desirable one.

Accepting clients who want to work on weight loss also gives us the opportunity to discuss feminist views about weight, eating, and the pursuit of beauty and thinness. Such discussions can be the first step towards the development of feelings of personal empowerment and the moderation of weight loss goals.

THE CASE AGAINST WEIGHT LOSS COUNSELING

No matter what the philosophy of the therapist, no matter what feminist conversations occur during the therapy sessions, taking on a client for weight loss counseling reinforces the cultural stereotypes and implies the therapist's acceptance of the beauty and fitness cults. By congratulating the client on weight loss, consoling her when she gains or remains the same, and urging her to change her food choices and eating style, the therapist is modeling fat oppression and suggesting that to be "good" her clients must follow her directions.

Fat women have often been told they are fat because they are "bad, wrong, and out of control" (Brown, 1987) and standard behavior therapy techniques for weight loss can be seen as supporting the opinion that fat women are responsible for their weight. Suggestions such as eat only when you are hungry, do not eat in response to emotions, plan your meals ahead of time, and make the best food choices lead to new ways to feel guilty (Brown, 1987) when clients cannot meet their goals.

Therapists often warn their clients not to use food as a reward, a suggestion which does not take into account that many women still do not have access to other "more appropriate" rewards (Brown, 1987). It is common for therapists to address the fact that women are often so busy giving to others that they do not take time out for themselves. We urge our clients to find the time to relax and to nurture themselves, and yet we deny the fact that feeding is an important part of self-nurturance (Brown, 1985), especially when there may be few other forms of self-nurturance available.

Even referring to our clients as "overweight" suggests that there is a correct and obtainable weight (Brown, 1985) and thus reinforces the stereotype of out of control people who are responsible for their weight. Recent physiological research has supported the existence of a genetic set point for weight (Mrosovsky & Sherry, 1980; Sims & Horton, 1968) and individual differences in metabolic activity (Keesey, 1980).

In addition, experiments demonstrating that insulin release can be classically conditioned (Woods et al., 1977; Wiley & Leveille, 1970) and that insulin can be released in some people when they see or smell food (Rodin, 1976) suggests that we have a limited amount of behavioral control over our weight. Encouraging our clients to do the impossible is neither feminist nor therapeutic. The fact that so many people deny these physiological mechanisms is testament to the morality our culture has assigned to weight and to the strength of fat oppression in our society.

More important for our clients than encouraging them to engage in a battle they will probably lose is to work instead on enhancing self-esteem and self-acceptance and increasing feelings of personal power. Several writers (Orbach, 1978; Brown, 1985) have pointed out that fat itself can be empowering. Reasons for rejecting cultural norms and supporting diversity of appearance should be discussed. The positive aspects of weight and the physiological processes which are programmed to maintain it should be explained. Clients can be encouraged to appreciate the freedom that accepting their weight can bring; it's liberating to give up those obsessions. Think of the time and energy we'll save by never weighing ourselves or counting our calories again!

CONCLUSION

Should feminist therapists do weight loss counseling? After setting forth the arguments for and against such counseling, it seems clear to me that the answer should be "no." And yet, I find myself unwilling to state that I have resolved never to do weight loss work again. I keep wondering about the client for whom weight loss might help to produce a genuine improvement in a medical condition and about the client who would desert the feminist therapist in favor of some drastic weight loss program. Perhaps a more honest answer is "rarely" or "hardly ever."

Although the answer may seem clearer in cases where the desired loss is for cosmetic reasons than when it is for medical reasons, I believe that each case requires an individual ethical decision. In reaching such a decision therapists must keep in mind the problem of fat oppression. Ask yourself whether you are in favor of weight loss counseling because of your own preference for thinness (Brown, 1985). Remember that there is no consensus on the amount of weight necessary to pose a health risk. When physicians refer their patients to us for weight loss counseling, we should consider whether the referral may be made because of the physicians' own attitudes toward fatness.

As Susie Orbach (1978) pointed out, "fat is a feminist issue." It is an issue not just for fat women, but for thin ones, and for therapists of all shapes and sizes whose clients ask for weight loss advice. We have a lot of thinking and talking to do before we reach a consensus on this one.

NOTE

1. The medical literature on the relationship of weight and health has been criticized (Rothblum, 1988) for two major research design flaws. First, there is no control for dieting despite the fact that some evidence suggests that dieting itself can lead to health risks (Brownell, 1980; Ernsberger, 1985). One can assume that most of the fat subjects in these studies were dieting at the time of the study or had recently been dieting; this results in a serious confounding of variables. Second, there is no control for socioeconomic status despite the fact that members of lower socioeconomic groups are more likely to be fat than members of higher socioeconomic groups (Moore, Stunkard, & Srole, 1962). Thus, the thin subjects in these studies may also be better educated, earning higher incomes, and receiving better medical care (Rothblum, 1988) than the fat subjects, again, a serious confounding of variables.

REFERENCES

Ballou, M., & Gabalac, N. W. (1985). *A feminist position on mental health.* Springfield, IL: Charles C Thomas.

Brown, L. S. (1985). Women, weight, and power: Feminist theoretical and therapeutic issues. *Women & Therapy, 4*(1), 61-71.

Brown, L. S. (1987). Lesbians, weight, and eating: New analyses and perspective. In Boston Lesbian Psychologies Collective, *Lesbian psychologies: Explorations & challenges.* (pp. 294-309). Chicago: University of Illinois Press.

Brownell, K. (1988). Yo-yo dieting. *Psychology Today,* pp. 20-23.

Editorial. (1987). Diabetes, diet, and exercise. *American Family Physician, 36*(3), 102-103.

Eichenbaum, L., & Orbach, S. (1983). *Understanding women: A feminist psychoanalytic approach.* New York: Basic Books.

Ernsberger, P. (1985). The death of dieting. *American Health, 4,* 29-33.

Fitzgerald, F. T. (1981). The problem of obesity. *Annual Review of Medicine, 32,* 221-231.

Freedman, R. (1986). *Beauty bound.* Lexington, MA: Lexington Books.

Keesey, R. E. (1980). A set point analysis of the regulation of body weight. In A. J. Stunkard (Ed.), *Obesity.* (pp. 144-165). Philadelphia: Saunders.

Keys, A. (1980). Overweight, obesity, coronary heart disease and mortality. *Nutrition Review, 38,* 297-307.

Moore, M. E., Stunkard, A., & Srole, L. (1962). Obesity, social class, and mental illness. *Journal of American Medical Association, 181,* 138-142.

Mrosovsky, N., & Sherry, D. F. (1980). Animal anorexias. *Science, 207,* 837-842.

Orbach, S. (1978). *Fat is a feminist issue.* New York: Berkeley Books.

Rodin, J. (1976). The role of perception of internal and external signals on regulation of feeding in overweight and nonobese individuals. In T. Silverstone (Ed.), *Appetite and food intake.* (pp. 265-283). Berlin: Life Sciences Research Report 2.

Rodin J., Silberstein, L., & Striegel-Moore, R. (1985). Woman and weight: A normative discontent. In *Nebraska symposium on motivation.* (pp. 267-304). Lincoln: University of Nebraska Press.

Rothblum, E. D. (1988). *Women and weight: Fad and fiction.* Manuscript submitted for publication.

Sims, E. A., & Horton, E. S. (1968). Endocrine and metabolic adaptation to obesity and starvation. *American Journal of Clinical Nutrition, 21,* 1455-1470.

Wiley, J. H., & Leveille, G. A. (1970). Significance of insulin in the metabolic adaptation of rats to meal ingestion. *Journal of Nutrition, 100,* 1073-1080.

Woods, S. C., Vasselli, J. R., Kaestner, E., Szakmary, G. A., Milburn, P., & Vitiello, M. V. (1977). Conditioned insulin secretion and meal feeding in rats. *Journal of Comparative and Physiological Psychology, 91,* 128-133.

Fat Acceptance Therapy (F.A.T.): A Non-Dieting Group Approach to Physical Wellness, Insight and Self-Acceptance

Susan Tenzer

SUMMARY. Group support can address the fat woman's unique plight and help raise her self-esteem. It can liberate her from a sense of powerlessness and worthlessness which is continually reinforced, especially if she has been fat since childhood. Her liberation begins with an understanding about why she cannot lose weight. The therapist must be informed about the physiology of adiposity, and appreciate the reality of a fat existence in this society and the damage it wrecks on a client's sense of self.

I am a fat woman. I am also a therapist specializing in eating disorders. When asked how I, as a fat woman, can treat anorexia, bulimia and obesity, I answer, "How could I not?" After hundreds of diets and thousands of dollars I am still fat. After years and years of oppression, I have let myself be free. The peace is overwhelming. This is the basis for fat acceptance therapy.

I was not fat as a child but as I watched my mother's fleshy body unfold out of her binding and restrictive girdles, a message, profound and lasting, became clear to me — FAT HURTS! It was an

---

Susan Tenzer, MA, CCMHC, NCC, is a certified clinical mental health counselor and founder/director of the Eating Disorder Treatment Center of the Lehigh Valley, Allentown, PA. In addition to being a specialist in the treatment of anorexia nervosa and bulimia, Mrs. Tenzer is a very active member of the National Association To Advance Fat Acceptance (NAAFA). She is currently on their Crisis Committee, chaired the Name Change Committee and lectures frequently on fat activism and fat acceptance.

object of derision and shame. No one (especially my father) would accept it.

When I reached puberty and my own body started to "blossom," my fears were confirmed. How would I ever live with this abundant and unfamiliar body? Even as a cheerleader and a 120 pound college student, I hated my body. That's when I discovered that starving would make it perfect. That revelation led me into sixteen years of amphetamine addiction. My successes were measured in diets that worked. Like the girdles that bound and restricted my mother, my weight gains held me hostage. However, my anger kept me from drowning. As the disgust with my body started to subside, a deeper, more encompassing, deliberate and conscious anger emerged. Why did I have to live this way? Why was there such a big price to pay for being thin? Why couldn't people accept me? Why couldn't I accept myself? I began to question the integrity of diet doctors, advertising, well-meaning friends who were "concerned for my health" and my own family. For years they had seen me high on pills and diets followed by the "crash" of the weight gains and the self-esteem. It was my body, I had to reclaim it. In the process of embracing it, there emerged a new and different emotion — grief. A time of mourning began for the diet that would inevitably fail and for the body that would never be thin. The journey from guilt to acceptance to celebration was a lengthy one. It came from therapy, a great deal of support and a wealth of knowledge.

The fat woman who enters my office for therapy usually has none of the above.

As her therapist, my goal is to instill in her a sense of esteem and worth as a fat woman and challenge, perhaps for the first time, her destructive and relentless attempts to be thin. It is in her best interest to see why dieting, a process which likely has added to the fat she carries (Bennett & Gurin, 1982) has been a preoccupation for much of her life. These realizations precede her readiness for fat acceptance therapy.

Through the process of therapy, we work through her intense feelings of anger and rage which have been repressed perhaps since childhood, perpetuating feelings of powerlessness, ineffectiveness and victimization.

UNDERSTANDING SETPOINT

The "setpoint" is an internal control system dictating how much fat a person should carry (Bennett & Gurin, 1982). Its physiology is only partly understood, yet it is almost universally acknowledged as a crucial determinant of adiposity by scientists in this field. Genetically, some individuals have a higher setting for fat than others (Bennett & Gurin, 1982).

If an organism is threatened with loss of nourishment — through a severe diet, for instance — the most "primitive" memory of feast and famine is awakened on the cellular level and the metabolism becomes much more efficient with calories and more vigilant at hoarding fat (Bennett & Gurin, 1982).

I have witnessed a dramatic illustration of setpoint firsthand with my cat who weighed seven pounds. She wandered away and was lost for about two months during which time she had lost half of her body weight. Following her rescue we noticed she no longer ate like a normal cat — taking a little food from its dish now and then. This cat ate voraciously. She ate everything in her dish immediately and continued to forage for more.

My cat did not "lack will power." She was not depressed and she did not have emotional problems. She was hungry and her body, with a setpoint driven up by near-starvation, knew what it needed. Six months following her ordeal she weighed 12 pounds and was considered clinically obese. Her body became well-padded to deal with the next disaster. In her case, that would be getting lost in the woods again.

In the fat woman's case, it could be the next diet.

Keys' study, "The Biology Of Human Starvation" (Keys et al., 1950) empirically studied dieting and refeeding. Thirty-six non-obese healthy men were observed during three months of normal eating, six months of semi-starvation (1,750 calories a day, or approximately half of their usual amount), and three months of refeeding. Though not approaching the level of starvation, they did follow the regime of any radical dieter and lost an average of 25 percent of their body weight, which is also the criteria for anorexia nervosa (American Psychiatric Association, 1980).

During the diet their lives focused increasingly and obsessively on food. Their metabolic rate dropped by 40 percent (Keys et al., 1950).

Their behavior, however, during refeeding was even more demonstrative for the therapist counseling fat people. They were unable to experience satiety regardless of the amount of food consumed. After an average of nine months, their appetites stabilized and they consumed normal amounts again (Keys et al., 1950). Every subject in the experiment eventually returned to his starting weight (setpoint). However, if the dieting had been repeated they would eventually go beyond that weight and establish a higher setpoint.

Their experience has not been replicated experimentally. But its results have been duplicated repeatedly in the lives of fat women.

FAT OPPRESSION

When I ask my clients why they believe their diets have failed, they usually blame themselves and their lack of will power. They see it as a repeated, personal failure. Many of these women have accomplished astonishing feats of self-denial. They hate themselves even while their self-starvation has unwittingly propelled the very mechanism that increases fat to prevent starvation (Garner & Garfinkel, 1985).

When she understands and believes the concept of setpoint and metabolism, the fat woman can finally ease that blame away from herself. When she sees dieting as a part of the problem, she stops the refeeding bingeing behavior that follows with its attendant self-hatred. Somewhere in the process of learning about setpoint, she realizes the futility of yet another diet.

No one knew these concepts when I was struggling with my weight. The insults from others and the loathing from myself was very destructive. The stigmatization, however, hasn't changed for fat because it is thought to be under voluntary control (Schoenfielder & Wieser, 1983). "Well-meaning" liberals still find it acceptable to intimidate, ridicule and judge us. Distaste for fat conveys a sense of aesthetic superiority in this society. Fat people are told they take up too much space. Facilities for people with disabilities are mandatory in most places. But for a fat woman a great deal of daily energy is spent trying to avoid embarrassment. She does not want to draw verbal comment from strangers. She wants to be sure that she can fit into the booth at McDonald's. She knows that if the room temperature feels normal to others, it will make her perspire visibly. She must reserve a seat in the front of the plane because the little tables on the other seats won't open in front of her. She fears losing her luggage because her clothes cannot be readily replaced. If someone picks her up in a smaller car, she may not be able to get in (Schoenfielder & Wieser, 1983). Personal classified ads request "slim" or "slender" women.

One of my worst recent experiences was at a parent/teacher conference. The desks were attached to the seats and one look told me I wouldn't fit. The insensitivity of the teacher was apparent as she spoke to me sitting at her desk while I stood uncomfortably for the entire conference. Incidentally, now I always request a straight chair when I schedule a school conference.

Social disapproval of fat has been reinforced by an assumption that greater body fat is harmful to health (Ernsberger & Haskew, 1987). This was exemplified in the 1985 NIH Consensus Development Conference Statement, "Health Implications Of Obesity" (Ernsberger & Haskew, 1987). It stated that anyone 20 percent over ideal weight is at risk for various disorders (Ernsberger & Haskew, 1987). By this description, the woman weighing more than 200 pounds is killing herself and anyone who helps her accept fat is abetting a suicide.

Less than two years later, a major rebuttal to this analysis was issued. In their report, "Rethinking Obesity," Ernsberger and Haskew (1987), consider factors such as the effects of dieting as a major health risk. They looked at so-called "obesity-related" diseases and the mistaken evidence qualifying the conclusion that fat alone is the causative factor. This report is essential reading for anyone who is involved with fat people, especially those badgering someone to diet "for her own good."

The fact is that fat people do not eat more than thin people, on the average (Garner & Garfinkel, 1985). It has been difficult for the scientific community to concur that this is what the data supports (Wooley & Wooley, 1984) because they have been brainwashed to believe that fat people have been gluttonous and dishonest about how much they actually eat.

I remember the incessant record keeping about what I ate. I also remember the futility of trying to convince my doctor that I wasn't lying. "You must be cheating," he said. I hated that word. It made me feel guilty and vulnerable. The weigh-ins caused me to become compliant and defiant. Somewhere deep inside of me, I knew I would have answers some day. And when I found them, no one would ever shame me again.

STARTING THE GROUP

For decades, fat women have been joining one another in diet clubs to lose weight. Typically, these groups provide enthusiastic support for the woman who is chiselling at her weight; a sense of failure for the woman who can't; and little acknowledgment that 90 percent of weight lost is regained within two years (Schwartz, 1982).

Group support can address the fat woman's unique plight and help raise her self-esteem. It can liberate her from the sense of worthlessness that is reinforced continually, and has caused real damage to her, especially if she has been fat since childhood. Her liberation begins with an understanding about why her body so vehemently defends its "set" weight. As her therapist, I am knowledgeable of the physiological aspects of weight and empathetic to the reality of being fat in a thin-obsessed society.

The setting for the group requires common sense anticipation of the fat woman's needs. Chairs must be wide, sturdy and not too high because the client cannot cross her legs. The room must be cool. And if stairs are involved, there should be an elevator.

GROUP DISCUSSION

Addressing size discrimination in the group is the first step in building a safe environment. They are all there because they share pain, memories and anger. Most of the participants have had some individual therapy and they are screened before joining the group. They have usually been enlightened as to the physiology of weight.

The first session generally consists of introductions and the sharing of histories of dieting. This can be a source of embarrassment but usually it eases the tension and creates bonding. It is also an opportunity to share myself. This self-disclosure removes the "me" versus "them" barriers. We are even able to laugh about the diets, the gimmicks and the multibillion dollar industry that "lives off the fat of the land."

In subsequent sessions, the history of being fat is the most critical part in discussing the origins of their pain and oppression. This is usually more profound in the participants who were always fat. In their formative years when they should have been building their self-esteem and egos, they were badly damaged, sometimes by the people they trusted the most—their parents.

WHAT IS FAT ACCEPTANCE?

The professionally led group can bring its participants to another level of behavior and cognition. It can help them change from victims to self-actualized people who have the ability to choose. Growth, as usual, is measured in slow, uneven changes.

Some of the groups in which I participated as a client were confrontive and rigid. I was told on several occasions that there was a thin person inside of me trying to emerge. When I questioned the validity of that, I was reminded that I was too angry and outspoken. No one understood.

My group has a right to its anger. Their perceptions change and those who have episodes of compulsive eating notice that it happens when they are coming off diets, diets that no one could possibly stick to. They see that the people who urged them to live on 800 calories a day for a year could no more do that than they could hold their breath for ten minutes.

They look at the percentage of people who fail at weight loss. They look at all the plans and diets that didn't work. They stop blaming their lack of will power. These women are anything but weak, lazy and uncontrolled. They need to see that in order to recognize their potential.

Reclaiming our bodies is paramount to fat acceptance. We are consumers and we patronize restaurants, clothing shops and doctors' offices. A doctor, dealing with his or her own distaste for fat or ignorant of the physiology involved, can cause a lot of damage to a fat person (NAAFA, Inc., 1987). We talk about ways to handle these problems by focusing on consumer rights.

Doctors tend to blame everything on fat (Ernsberger & Haskew, 1987). Fat women get blamed and criticized and handed 1,000 calorie diets and told to "use your will power." A fat woman can be a paying customer for this abuse, or she can discuss it as a problem with the doctor. She can point out that her blood pressure is higher at the medical clinic, as has been documented, because of the anxiety the physician evokes about her fat. She can seek a physician who is more sophisticated about her health and care.

As the group progresses, I look for greater confidence and better coping with social disapproval. Some of the changes that become evident are: greater confidence about going out, eating in public, dressing more attractively and asserting her right to respect (NAAFA, Inc., 1987).

What we really learn to handle is relationships, especially intimate relationships. With the greatest of luck, these women have discovered friends who we call F.A.'s or Fat Admirers (NAAFA, Inc., 1987). If a woman can accept her size, but her loved one cannot, the group supports her in accommodating that opinion for the sake of a relationship she likes, or choosing to end the relationship for the damage it does to her.

At this point, the group is dealing with issues far beyond "dieting." There are enormous rewards for a therapist who sees this kind of growth. An average fat woman has developed such personal strengths, just from enduring her plight, that once she taps those resources on her own behalf, she changes rapidly. The change is evident, despite what she weighs (NAAFA, Inc., 1987).

When a woman drops the very notion of dieting and refeeding, she begins the more enjoyable process of listening to her body and its needs. She starts to eat reasonably and in response to hunger (Schwartz, 1982). She may also decide to begin exercising. She is responding to her body's needs despite the comments she gets. It is an act of friendship toward herself.

CONCLUSION

Fat people carry an enormous burden. It is not the burden of massive bodies, or insatiable appetites, but the burden of oppression the culture forces upon them. They are weighed down not by their weight, but by the force of hatred, contempt and pity, amusement and revulsion. Fat bodies are invaded by comments, measured with hatred, pathologized by fear and diagnosed by ignorance . . . (Bull, 1987)

"Our task is for these women to learn to love and accept their fat bodies. They will then be free to feed and move and dress and honor it" (Bull, 1987).

In order to be free from conflict, a person must find acceptance or change. For 95 percent of the 30 million American women who wear size 16 or larger (NAAFA, Inc., 1987), dramatic weight change is not possible. Therefore, the best alternative is fat acceptance. I am grateful that I found that.

REFERENCES

American Psychiatric Association (1980). *Diagnostic and statistical manual of mental disorders* (3rd ed.). Washington, DC: APA.

Bennett, W., & Gurin, J. (1982). *The dieter's dilemma*. New York: Basic Books.

Bull, R. (1987, April). Challenging the myth: Some facts on fat. *Matrix*, 3.

Ernsberger, P., & Haskew, P. (1987). Rethinking obesity. *The Journal of Obesity and Weight Regulation*, 6.

Garner, D., & Garfinkel, P. (1985). *Handbook of psychotherapy for anorexia nervosa and bulimia*. New York: The Guilford Press.

Keys, A., Brozek, J., Henschel, A., Mickelsen, O., & Taylor, H. L. (1950). *The biology of human starvation*. Minneapolis: University of Minnesota Press.

NAAFA, Inc. (1987). *NAAFA workbook—a complete study guide*. Bellerose, NY: Author.

Schoenfielder, L., & Wieser, B. (1983). *Shadow on a tightrope*. Iowa City, IA: Aunt Lute Book Company.

Schwartz, R. (1982). *Diets don't work*. Galveston, TX: Breakthru Publishing.

Wooley, S. C., & Wooley, O. W. (1984). Should obesity be treated at all? In A. J. Stunkard and E. Stellar (Eds.), *Eating and its disorders*. New York: Raven Press.

The Role of Stigmatization
in Fat People's Avoidance
of Physical Exercise

Jaclyn Packer

SUMMARY. The stigmatization that fat people face discourages them from engaging in physical exercise as a means of maintaining health; social factors (e.g., fear of being ridiculed by others; inaccessible exercise equipment, clothing and facilities) negatively influence fat people's motivation to exercise, and has an especially strong impact on women. The relationship between exercise and weight loss is discussed, and the assumption that fat people can become thin through physical exercise will be critiqued. Suggestions are made for improving the group exercise situation for fat people, and the need for further research is discussed.

Physical exercise has been shown to be one of the most important factors related to people's health (Dishman & Dunn, 1986, Wetzler & Cruess, 1985). In addition to contributing to health, exercise is a social/recreational activity and may also contribute to feelings of psychological well-being and improvement of self-esteem (Dishman & Dunn, 1986, Stern, 1984). Exercise should be an activity that people of all ages, weights, body types, backgrounds and abilities can participate in. Exercise may make an especially strong contribution to the health of those who are heavier because fat people appear to be at higher risk for diseases associated with lack of exercise; ironically, social factors make opportunities to exercise least accessible to them. This paper will discuss the ways in which the stigmatization of fatness in our society (Allon, 1982, Millman,

Jaclyn Packer is a doctoral candidate in the Social/Personality Psychology program at the Graduate Center of the City University of New York. She is the author of several articles on disability and on issues affecting women.

49

1980, Wadden & Stunkard, 1985) discourages vast numbers of people, especially women, from exercising as a means of maintaining health, and will also critique the assumption that fat people can become thin through exercise.

Physical exercise for fat people is often regarded primarily as a means to become thin; because of this, exercise is often overlooked as an important means of maintaining and improving health when not connected with a weight-loss effort. Discussions regarding the questionable long-term success of dieting have been developed elsewhere (Bennett & Gurin, 1982, Ernsberger & Haskew, 1987). Literature on weight loss indicates that very few people who try to reduce their weight for any significant length of time will be successful (Wooley & Wooley, 1979). Because dieting is not likely to work, and may have ill effects on health, it is important to promote exercise as a means of health maintenance in the absence of weight loss. Fat people should be encouraged to engage in exercising for their health; factors that keep fat people from exercising need to be identified and attempts need to be made to eliminate barriers. Although this paper will be focusing on the issue of health, one should also keep in mind that these barriers to exercise also keep fat people from experiencing the fun of exercise and sports in social/recreational contexts, and from obtaining the benefits of psychological well-being that people get from exercising.

This paper makes the assumption that physical exercise will have a positive effect on the health of fat people; it is important to note, however, that while virtually all studies concerning fat people and exercise have focused on whether or how well exercise promotes weight loss, few studies have concerned themselves with whether conventional exercise is actually healthy for those at higher weights. It is important that such studies be conducted; however it is unlikely that this will be a prominent research focus until there is less emphasis placed on the use of exercise for weight loss.

THE RELATIONSHIP BETWEEN EXERCISE
AND WEIGHT LOSS

Until quite recently, most of the literature on fatness concerned the problem of how to get fat people to become normative-sized, or to explain the ways in which fat people were psychologically different from those of normative weight.* A number of studies have shown that fat people do not exercise as much as normative weight people, and indicate that this may be a contributing factor to their being fat (Johnson, Burke & Mayer, 1956, Chirico & Stunkard, 1960, Bullen, Reed & Mayer, 1964). Note that because fat people weigh more, they are actually performing more work when carrying out equivalent movements to normative weight people. This should be taken into consideration when comparing physical activity between fat people and others (Wooley & Wooley, 1979). Also, because fat people are stigmatized, physical activity studies may be unduly influenced by fat people's feelings of self-consciousness or embarrassment at being watched during sports and other exercise (Allon, 1982).

Many people advocate the notion that if people simply use up, through physical activity, more calories than they eat, they will eventually become thin. The biggest problem with this concept is that many people maintain extremely high weights despite low-calorie intake and normal activity levels; the amount of time that one would have to devote to exercise, in order to reduce down from an extremely high body weight, would drastically alter a person's normal lifestyle. According to many experts on exercise, in order for most people to be physically fit, they have to spend twenty to thirty minutes doing aerobic exercise, three to five times per week. Therefore, at most, people would typically need to spent 2 1/2 hours a week exercising. While it may be difficult to find the time, many people are able to do just this. But take the case of a person well above "ideal" weight. According to Katahn (1984), most people who are 50 pounds over "ideal" would only have to exercise approximately 45 minutes a day, 7 days a week, and they will get down to a normative weight. Presumably, then, a person who is 100 pounds over normative weight would only have to devote an hour and a half a day, 7 days per week. And a person 200 pounds above the norm? Three hours a day, 7 days a week. If one adds on to this the amount of time it takes to get to the place of exercise activity,

*The term "normative weight" will be used in preference to the popular term "normal weight" to refer to those who fit the cultural norm for appropriate size. According to Ritenbaugh (1982), the statistical norm (average) weight of the population is actually *much higher* than the cultural norm.

change into appropriate exercise clothing, and do necessary warming up/winding down exercises, the person might need to spend 4 1/2 hours or more per day (31 1/2 hours per week — almost a full-time job!) pursuing their ideal weight through exercise. Certainly, if a person 200 pounds above the ideal were to devote four or five hours a day, every day, to physical exercise, he/she would most likely eventually become normative weight; however *at what cost*? The person's life would be one with little time for pleasure, leisure, family or normal life obligations. Perhaps this is the reason that of the tiny minority of people who lose weight and keep it off for any significant length of time, many are people who are employed in the weight-loss industry (exercise instructors, diet counselors) and who therefore focus their entire lives (including their jobs) on weight loss. Now that we are beginning to recognize the futility of spending our lives dieting (since few people really do lose weight permanently) we are now being encouraged to literally spend our lives exercising. Women in our society typically have even less leisure time than men have; therefore the notion that all fat people need to do is get "enough" exercise is particularly oppressive to women.

The empirical evidence on whether exercise aids weight loss is mixed. Bennett and Gurin (1982) believe that exercise is the *only* effective way to lower one's weight "set-point" and lose weight. They maintain that "an active body is set to be thinner than an inactive one." However, they admit that it is a slow way to lose weight and is unlikely to produce dramatic changes in weight for everyone. Patton (1982) believes that exercise is important for everyone, but that it should not be looked at as a means to get thin — only to get healthy. An annotated bibliography on physical activity and obesity (Fleming & Frederiksen, 1981) cites fifteen studies that focus on exercise as a means of weight control. Less than half the cited studies showed weight loss as a result of physical exercise. The remaining studies showed either no weight loss or had insufficient data. Several of the studies found a decrease in body fat although no change in total body weight was found. Note that the results of these studies include only those subjects who did not drop out; attrition is a pervasive problem in this type of research (Geleibter, 1982), and social factors are rarely mentioned as a reason for the high drop out rate.

Mayer (1983) questions why researchers don't ask whether fat people are less active because they are underfed, as a result of dieting, and therefore lack energy. Others have also pointed out the lack of energy that results from dieting as a factor in decreased physical activity (Bennett & Gurin, 1982, Wooley, Wooley & Dyrenforth, 1979). Because fat people are stigmatized, and are often the brunt of verbal abuse because of their size, Mayer (1983) further questions where fat people would be able to exercise, free from ridicule. According to Ernsberger (1982), "The harassment and ridicule that fat people are subject to, make it less likely that they will swim, jog or bicycle. The harassment that comes from just walking down the street may lead some fat people to lead sedentary lives." Many other factors appear to be operating which discourage fat people from exercising. It will be difficult to ascertain, through research, whether physical exercise promotes weight loss and/or contributes to health among fat people until social and physical environments exist in which fat people will feel comfortable exercising.

SOCIAL FACTORS INFLUENCING
FAT PEOPLE'S AVOIDANCE OF EXERCISE

Some of the reasons why exercise is not as accessible to fat people as it is to others will be examined. It will be proposed that this situation can be changed by encouraging fat people to exercise for the purpose of maintaining health, rather than focusing on weight loss, and by setting up more conducive exercise environments.

Many health problems that are usually associated with obesity may actually be caused by lack of exercise (Ernsberger, 1982), and many can be prevented or alleviated through exercise (Geleibter, 1982, Lampman, Santinga & Savage, 1982). The connection between fat people's sedentary lifestyles and their health problems will remain unclear, until they are given an opportunity to engage in exercise to the same extent as other people.

There is little in the research literature that examines why fat people do not exercise, and virtually none of the literature addresses the issue of how to arrange a physically and psychologically comfortable exercise environment that will motivate and encourage exercise among fat people. While numerous studies on exercise for weight control state that large numbers of subjects dropped out or did not comply (Geleibter, 1982), reasons are rarely speculated upon. Occasionally the issue of motivation is mentioned. More rarely, the issue of exercise being a more difficult task for a fat person is mentioned (Rodin, 1982, Dishman, 1982). Social factors affecting fat people are virtually ignored in the issue of compliance to exercise programs. According to Leventhal and Hirschman (1982), while situational factors may cause non-compliance to health regimens, they are often overlooked in favor of blaming the person. This is certainly the case with fat people, whose often sedentary lifestyles are blamed on laziness.

There are many more factors which prevent fat people from exercising than are usually addressed in the literature; each of these reasons is ultimately related to the stigma that people face in this culture when they feel they are above society's norm for weight. Some or all of these factors operate in each of the three most popular exercise domains (on public streets, in exercise groups/clubs, in one's own home) and impact on fat people's motivation to engage in or continue exercising. These reasons include:

- the belief that dieting is much more important for health than exercising;
- the belief that attractiveness is more important than health;
- fear of ridicule from others;
- difficulty in keeping up with others or looking awkward;
- environmental/attitudinal inaccessibility of exercise facilities;
- fear of physical injury or harm;
- difficulty in finding exercise clothing that fits;
- lack of financial resources.

While attitudes toward fat people are extremely negative, these attitudes appear to affect women more than men. Because appearance is much more critical for women than men, fatness is a much worse problem for women (Allon, 1982, Millman, 1980, Wooley, Wooley & Dyrenforth, 1979); therefore, most of the factors that prevent fat people from exercising will probably have a stronger influence on women. Compounding the greater stigma that fat women face is the fact that, in general, women (fat or thin) are not encouraged as much as men to be active and physically fit.

Belief That Dieting Is More Important for Health

While most research on exercise shows its positive effects on health, the research on dieting is equivocal at best; despite this, the public is constantly exposed to mass media messages about the desirability of dieting; this far exceeds people's exposure to positive messages about exercise. Physicians tend to put more emphasis on dieting than on exercise for their fat patients. D'Amelio (1976) reports that while 65% of physicians prescribe low-calorie diets for patients they consider to be "seriously overweight," and 75% prescribe weight-loss drugs to at least some of their patients, only 11% advise them to get more exercise. Only a short time ago, doctors believed that exercise was actually *detrimental* to a dieter's weight-loss attempts (Stuart & Davis, 1972). Many fat people are therefore more motivated to put energy into dieting than into exercise, for health purposes. According to Ernsberger (1982), people who are fat often feel that they are doomed to an early death — since they are fat they *must* be unhealthy, and therefore they see no reason to bother to attempt to improve or maintain their health. If they are not actively dieting, many fat people feel there is no need to bother exercising.

Belief That Attractiveness Is More Important Than Health

Fat people are usually not encouraged to exercise for health unless it is also to achieve a thin ideal. In fact, many people are willing to put their lives in jeopardy in order to lose weight, as evidenced by the epidemic of anorexia and bulimia in this country. Mayer (1983) quotes a fat woman as saying "I wish I could get cancer or some other wasting disease, so I could die thin." The idea of looking "attractive" (or at the very least not stigmatized) is much more salient to people (particularly women) than maintaining their health. This is not surprising, considering that people in our society are constantly being exposed to a barrage of messages which equate fatness with unattractiveness. While we are also exposed to messages equating fatness with ill-health, these are not as pervasive as those related to appearance.

Despite the very high death rate involved with weight-loss surgery, 30 to 50 thousand people elect this surgery every year (Ernsberger, 1984), so that even if they give up on their health, they can, at least, be thin. If the true objective of weight-loss surgery were to improve people's health, one would expect that fat men would be twice as likely to undergo this surgery since they are at the much greater risk of illness from obesity. However, the fact is that 80 to 90% of weight-loss surgery is done to women (Ernsberger, 1984).

Much of our society's preoccupation with slimness has more to do with attractiveness than health. A recent study by Hayes and Ross (1987) demonstrated that many people are motivated to engage in healthy behaviors out of their concern for their appearance; the authors suggest that the recent trend toward exercise and physical fitness is partly motivated by people's attempts to conform to a smaller ideal body size, especially for women. They conclude that when good health practices and appearance norms coincide, women benefit; but if current fashion dictated poor health practices, women might then engage in those practices for the sake of attractiveness. Garner (1984) states that society's recent emphasis on exercise and fitness is for women almost completely focused on their becoming thin. He feels that this emphasis affects not only fat women, but any woman who does not have the body of a slim high-fashion model. Many fat people feel that if they are not making a strong effort to diet, then exercising is a waste of time. Therefore, many people exercise *only* when they are also dieting.

Fear of Ridicule from Others

Many fat people have experienced being stared at and ridiculed by others while they exercise. This is especially true for exercise done on public streets, such as jogging or bicycle riding, but it also applies to exercising at health clubs. Exercise instructors often make disparaging comments about fatness, in order to "encourage" exercisers to keep at it. This is in spite of research showing that people are much more likely to comply in health situations when they feel they are respected and liked by the health care provider (Rodin & Janis, 1979, Stone, 1979). Dishman (1982) states that the types of social reinforcement displayed by other exercisers or exercise instructors affect people's exercise behaviors. Since many exercise instructors outwardly exhibit disdain toward fatness and fat people, it is not likely that many fat people will feel motivated to attend exercise classes. People who exercise in the privacy of their own home, in order to avoid public scrutiny, may fear ridicule from members of their own families. Additionally, there is evidence that people are much more likely to comply with and continue an exercise program when they are doing it as part of a group (Gwinup, 1975, Geleibter, 1982, Hanefeld, Zschornack & Weck, 1981), so "going it alone" is not a very viable alternative.

Difficulty in Keeping Up with Others or Looking Awkward

There is evidence that it is more difficult for a fat person to do various types of exercise than it is for those of normative weight (Dishmen, 1982, Rodin, 1982). Exercise programs often are not geared for persons who may be out of shape, or need to begin at a slower pace. According to Dwyer, Feldman and Mayer (1970), school physical education programs are aimed at fit children. Fat children are often inactive and feel clumsy; they need programs specially adapted for them. Certainly, a person (of any weight) who decides to begin a program of exercise will have a lot of trouble at the beginning. Fat people who decide to join a group or club often find themselves in a room full of people who are much slimmer than they are, and who appear to have little trouble keeping up with the class (partly because they weigh less, and partly because most of them have been exercising longer). This situation may lead to feelings of self-consciousness and possibly humiliation at not being able to keep up. In addition, the person may be presented with the challenge of attempting an exercise that is either physically impossible for them, or that will be physically unhealthy for them to perform (DuCoff & Cohen, 1980). Leventhal and Hirschman (1982) feel that health promotion groups should "focus attention on positive body sensations . . . ease of movement . . . and positive affect" in order to encourage people to engage in health promoting activities. However, there is usually little encouragement and great disincentive at an exercise club to attempt to tailor an exercise program to one's own individual physical needs. Dishman (1982) feels that a more individual program would lead to greater compliance, especially if some degree of choice is involved. In addition, he states that one's perception of having sufficient ability to perform exercise successfully is an important factor in a person's deciding to begin an exercise program. Because of the constant discouragement fat people face in the area of physical activity, it is difficult for them to gain confidence in their physical ability.

Environmental/Attitudinal Inaccessibility of Exercise Facilities

Some exercise environments are not physically accessible to many fat people. For example, exercise classes may be very crowded, leaving little space for a person to stand and move; exercise bicycles may have small seats which are extremely uncomfortable for larger people. In addition, many clubs have features which may add to a fat person's emotional discomfort, including scales prominently displayed, which project the message that weight loss is the purpose of being there, and walls covered with mirrors. Many fat people have reported that they actively avoid seeing their own reflections (Rand & Stunkard, 1978), so they might avoid exercise classes which are held in large areas surrounded by mirrors. In addition to the inaccessibility of the physical environment itself, fat people have actually been denied membership in exercise clubs because of their weight (Out of court settlement, 1986). Wadden and Stunkard (1985) maintain that the physical environment often limits fat people's mobility, constrains their opportunities for physical activity, and subjects them to humiliation. Ironically, this seems to be particularly true in environments that are intended for physical activity.

Fear of Physical Injury or Harm

As stated previously, fat people are often encouraged to do exercises which may be impossible for them or physically harmful. In addition, fat people may have an exaggerated sense of their own susceptibility to illness or heart attack because of the widespread belief that fatness causes poor health, and may feel they should not be engaging in exercise because of this. The public needs to become educated about the questionable causal link between fatness and ill health (Ernsberger & Haskew, 1987), and more research needs to be conducted on what types of exercise are safe and physically beneficial for fat people.

Difficulty in Finding Exercise Clothing That Fits

Until very recently, it was impossible to find many types of functional clothing in large sizes, particularly women's clothing. (This is in spite of the fact that over 30 percent of adult women in the United States wear a size 16 or larger, Ducoff & Cohen, 1980.) Large-size clothing manufacturers apparently didn't think that fat women exercised, because very little exercise clothing was ever available. Mayer (1983) mentions the lack of availability of large-size gym suits for fat high school students. Recently there has been a trend toward having more clothing available in larger sizes; however it is still difficult for very large women to find clothing and the large sizes tend to cost more money than clothing in smaller sizes (Riggs, 1983).

Lack of Financial Resources

A negative correlation between weight and socioeconomic-status has been found in several studies (Stunkard, D'Aquili, Fox & Filon, 1972, Goldblatt, Moore & Stunkard, 1965.) This relationship is especially strong for fat women (Weil, 1983). Goldblatt, Moore and Stunkard (1965) found that lower socioeconomic-status women were six times more likely to be fat compared to women of higher status. They also found that women who were upwardly mobile were much less likely to be fat than those who were downwardly mobile. Similar trends were found for men in their sample, but were much less marked.

Because of the lower socioeconomic-status of fat people (resulting, in part, from employment discrimination), chances are that they can least afford to buy exercise clothing and equipment or join health and exercise clubs. In addition, people who have more money may be able to gain leisure time, for example, by shifting chores and obligations to paid help; therefore, fat people, especially women, are less likely to have the luxury of having free time available to exercise.

Many of the points discussed above have been supported by data collected on a small sample of people attending a Weight Watchers class in New York City (N = 28). On a closed-ended questionnaire, clear differences emerged when subjects were split into two groups — those who had ever been 50 pounds or more over Weight Watchers' prescribed goal for the person (based on current medical recommendations), and those who had been 49 or less pounds over this goal at their highest weight. More subjects in the heavier group indicated that a reason they did not exercise was that they were unable to find exercise clothing that fit, or that they were not able to afford to join an exercise group. Items that most differentiated the two groups were those items involving fear of injury, feeling clumsy or awkward, difficulty exercising and embarrassment in front of others. Seventy-two percent of the heavier group said that embarrassment was a reason they had ever not exercised. Only 8% of the thinner group said it was ever a reason. Although the subjects felt strongly that exercise is important for good health, only half were currently exercising, and only a third were exercising the last time they were not dieting. Subjects also tended to exercise for much less time when they were not dieting.

Two-thirds of the sample indicated that not wanting to exercise alone was an important enough factor to keep them from exercising at all. Research has shown that the most successful involvement in exercise involves participation in groups. Therefore, it is most important to focus on changes that can be incorporated into group exercise environments. There should be special exercise classes offered just for fat people, in order to reduce feelings of self-consciousness; these classes might be held in rooms without mirrors and scales. There should be easier exercise classes offered for people (of all weight levels) who are not yet ready for an intense workout, or alternatively, people should be encouraged to exercise at their own pace until they are ready to do more. Exercise instructors should be educated so that they do not use fear of fat as a scare tactic to motivate their members. Exercise equipment should be adapted so that it is comfortable for larger people to use. More research needs to be conducted that focuses on whether such changes would increase participation, and how greater involvement in exercise activity affects the health status of fat people.

Therapists who work with fat clients must be aware of their own prejudices around the issue of weight, and must be careful not to assume that the difficulties a client experiences, such as strong feelings of self-consciousness around exercising, are a reflection of intrapsychic problems. The therapist should always consider first whether their fat client's feelings and behavior reflect a normal reaction to a hostile environment. Therapists can help their fat clients explore the ways in which the social environment contributes to their avoidance of exercise. Clients must be discouraged from internalizing blame for exercise avoidance; feelings that one is lazy or doesn't care about one's health should be dealt with in the client-therapist relationship. Clients should be encouraged to seek out alternatives to traditional exercise situations, where they can feel more comfortable engaging in exercise. Finally, therapists should promote the idea that exercise may be an enjoyable and healthful activity which is separate from the issue of weight loss.

Everyone deserves the right to be able to contribute as much as possible to their own emotional and physical well-being. Perhaps, through further research and through public education, some of the barriers that keep fat people from exercising can be eliminated. Only when these barriers are gone can this significant portion of the population be free to engage in an important and healthful activity that should be available to every human being.

REFERENCES

Allon, N. (1982). The stigma of overweight in everyday life. In B. Wolman (Ed.), *Psychological aspects of obesity: A handbook.* New York: Van Nostrand Reinhold Co.

Bennett, W., & Gurin, J. (1982). *The dieter's dilemma: Eating less and weighing more: The scientific case against dieting as a means of weight control.* New York: Basic Books, Inc.

Bullen, B.A., Reed, R.B., & Mayer, J. (1964). Physical activity of obese and non-obese adolescent girls, appraised by motion picture sampling. *Journal of Clinical Nutrition, 14,* 211-23.

Chirico, A.M., & Stunkard, A.J. (1960). Physical activity and human obesity. *New England Journal of Medicine, 263,* 935-940.

D'Amelio, N. (1976). How family doctors are treating their overweight patients. *Medical Times, 104*(12), 51-57.

Dishman, R.K. (1982). Compliance/adherence in health related exercise. *Health psychology, 1*, 237-267.

Dishman, R.K., & Dunn, A.L. (1986). Exercise adherence in children and youth: Implications for adulthood. In R.K. Dishman (Ed.), *Exercise adherence: Its impact on public health*. Champaign, IL: Human Kinetics Books.

DuCoff, J., & Cohen, S.C. (1980). *Making it big: A guide to health, success and beauty for the woman size 16 and over*. New York: Simon & Schuster.

Dwyer, J.T., Feldman, J.J., & Mayer, J. The social psychology of dieting. *Journal of Health and Social Behavior, 11*, 269-287.

Ernsberger, P. (1982). *Fat and health: What your doctor probably doesn't know*. New York: National Association to Aid Fat Americans.

Ernsberger, P. (1984). *Report on weight-loss surgery*. New York: National Association to Aid Fat Americans.

Ernsberger, P., & Haskew, P. (1987). Rethinking obesity: An alternative view of its health implications. *Journal of Obesity and Weight Regulation, 6*(2), 57-137.

Fleming, C., & Frederiksen, L. (1981). Physical activity and obesity: An annotated bibliography. *Catalog of Selected Documents in Psychology, 11*, 81.

Garner, D. (1984, August). *Sociocultural factors in anorexia nervosa and bulimia*. Public lecture at the meeting of the American Psychological Association, Toronto, Canada.

Geleibter, A. (1982). Exercise and obesity. In B. Wolman (Ed.), *Psychological aspects of obesity: A handbook*. New York: Van Nostrand Reinhold Co.

Goldblatt, P.B., Moore, M.E., & Stunkard, A.J. (1965). Social factors in obesity. *Journal of the American Medical Association, 192*(12), 97-102.

Gwinup, G. (1975). Effect of exercise alone on the weight of obese women. *Archives of Internal Medicine, 135*, 676.

Hanefeld, M., Zschornack, M., & Weck, M. (1982). Physical training in obese subjects: Selection, motivation, organization and follow-up problems. In R. Bjorntorp, M. Cairella, & A. Howard (Eds.), *Recent advances in obesity research, III*. London: John Libbey.

Hayes, D., & Ross, C.E. (1987). Concern with appearance, health beliefs and eating habits. *Journal of Health and Social Behavior, 28*(2), 120-130.

Johnson, M.L., Burke, B., & Mayer, J. (1956). Relative importance of inactivity and overeating in energy balance of obese high school girls. *American Journal of Clinical Nutrition, 4*, 37-44.

Katahn, M. (1984). *Beyond diet*. New York: Berkley Books.

Lampman, R.M., Santinga, J.T., & Savage, P.J. (1982). Effect of exercise training on glucose tolerance, insulin resistance and lipid metabolism in middle-aged men. In B. Wolman (Ed.), *Psychological aspects of obesity*. New York: Van Nostrand Reinhold Co.

Leventhal, H., & Hirschman, R.S. (1982). Social psychology and prevention. In

G. Sanders & J. Suls (Eds.), *Social psychology of health and illness*. Hillsdale, NJ: Erlbaum Associates.

Mayer, V. (1983). The fat illusion. In L. Shoenfelder & B. Wieser (Eds.), *Shadow on a tightrope*. Iowa City, IA: Aunt Lute Book Co.

Millman, M. (1980). *Such a pretty face: Being fat in America*. New York: Berkley Books.

Out of court settlement made in health spa lawsuit. (1986, August). *National Association to Aid Fat Americans (NAAFA) Newsletter*, p. 1.

Patton, S. (1982). *Stop dieting, start living*. New York: Dodd, Mead & Co., Inc.

Rand, C.R., & Stunkard, A.J. (1978). Obesity and psychoanalysis. *American Journal of Psychiatry, 135*(5), 547-551.

Riggs, C. (1983). Fat women and clothing. In L. Shoenfelder & B. Wieser (Eds.), *Shadow on a tightrope*. Iowa City, IA: Aunt Lute Book Co.

Ritenbaugh, C. (1982). Obesity as a culture-bound syndrome. *Culture, Medicine and Psychiatry, 6*(4), 347-361.

Rodin, J. (1982). Obesity: Why the losing battle? In B. Wolman (Ed.), *Psychological aspects of obesity*. New York: Van Nostrand Reinhold Co.

Rodin, J., & Janis, I.L. (1979). The social power of health care practitioners as agents of change. *Journal of Social Issues, 35*, 60-81.

Stern, J. (1984). Is obesity a disease of inactivity? In A.J. Stunkard & E. Stellar (Eds.), *Eating and its disorders*. New York: Raven Press.

Stone, G.C. (1979). Patient compliance and the role of the expert. *Journal of Social Issues, 35*, 34-59.

Stunkard, A.J., D'Aquili, E., Fox, S., & Filion, R.D.L. (1972). Influence of social class on obesity and thinness in children. *Journal of the American Medical Association, 221*, 579.

Stuart, R., & Davis, B. (1972). *Slim chance in a fat world: Behavioral control of obesity,*. Champaign, IL: Research Press.

Syme, S.L. (1978). Lifestyle intervention in clinic-based trials. *American Journal of Epidemiology, 108*, 87-91.

Wadden, T.A., & Stunkard, A.J. (February, 1985). *Adverse social and psychological consequences of obesity*. Paper presented at National Institutes for Health Consensus Development Conference on the "Health Implications of Obesity," Bethesda, MD.

Weil, W. (1983). The demographic characteristics of fatness and obesity. In B. Hansen (Ed.), *Controversies in obesity, volume 5*. New York: Praeger.

Wetzler, H.P., & Cruess, D.F. (1985). Self-reported physical health practices and health care utilization: Findings from the National Health Interview Survey. *American Journal of Public Health, 75*(11), 1329-1330.

Wooley, S.C., & Wooley, O.W. (1979). Obesity and women – I. A closer look at the facts. *Women's Studies International Quarterly, 2*, 69-79.

Wooley, S.C., Wooley, O.W., & Dyrenforth, S.R. (1979). Obesity and women – II. A neglected feminist topic. *Women's Studies International Quarterly, 2*, 81-92.

Fitness, Feminism and the Health of Fat Women

Pat Lyons

SUMMARY. As a fat woman all my life, in this paper I want to share my experience of turning self-hatred into self-love and healing. Combining principles and practices of feminism, wellness and sport psychology I returned, after many years' absence, to my childhood love of sports. I began to live a more healthy life despite never attaining my "ideal" weight. Sport and movement are fundamental ways for all women to learn to trust and enjoy their bodies and improve their health. But because of sexism women have not only been objectified and taught to focus on their appearance, but have been denied full access to sport and exercise opportunities. Beyond this basic problem shared with all women, fat women are ridiculed and made the objects of scorn in the standard fitness environment, particularly if they do not lose weight for their efforts. Therefore, because fat women have unique exercise needs that have been ignored, I co-authored, and will summarize here, *Great Shape: The First Exercise Guide for Large Women* (Arbor House/William Morrow, 1988, co-author, Debby Burgard). Finally, I'll address the issue of isolation, which occurs because of the social prejudice against fat people and can create physical and mental health problems. It is my intention to help create a world where we all live with self-respect and in vibrant good health, whatever our size.

I've been fat all of my life. I've suffered the blows society dishes out to those of us whose genetically determined bodies refuse to

Pat Lyons, RN, MA, has been a community health nurse and women's health advocate for over twenty years. She obtained her master's degree in psychology, emphasizing sport psychology and women's health, in 1984 at Sonoma State University. Former Director of Community Education and Health Promotion for Toiyabe Indian Health Project, Bishop, CA, she is now a health care consultant living in San Francisco, CA.

65

conform to "ideal" weight charts—a childhood full of "fatty-fatty-two-by-four" taunts, and later, discrimination in jobs, thin women talking about how disgusting they are because of five "extra" pounds (what must they think of me?) and men who said they'd love me more if I was thinner. During my twenties I dieted furiously—with the help of cigarettes, Tab, and speed—and indeed I lost weight. But I felt miserable and was depressed most of the time too, particularly when I inevitably gained the weight back. Little did I know then that 98% of all diets fail regardless of the slogans, food substitutes and guilt trips promoted by Weight Watchers and their ilk (Bennett & Gurin, 1982).

Year after year, I waited, hoped and prayed for the magic of willpower to descend from the heavens into my life and make me lastingly, finally thin. It didn't happen. As I yo-yoed up and down the scale I blamed my weight for all misery. People around me reinforced this idea by telling me I had such a pretty face, and if I would only lose weight I'd be happy. What I saw as repeated dieting failure only made me hate myself more, and turned my thoughts to suicide more than once.

When I was 31, a wise friend told me that before I could accept and love myself and live a happier life I had to learn to love my body. I thought she was nuts. How could I possibly learn to love this fat, embarrassing, humiliating body of mine? But despite my determined resistance, her words stayed with me. In the months after our conversation I realized that I could continue to be miserable or I could set out to enjoy, rather than endure my life, and maybe I could even learn to like myself. (It was still too early then to say "love" myself and mean it.) I was certainly ready to try something different to feel better. I was very tired of looking into the mirror and seeing tears slide down my cheeks.

In this article I'd like to share my process of turning self-hatred into self-love. I am fat and at 43 I am healthy and finally at peace with my body. I hope my experience can help therapists who are working with women agonizing about their weight. Millions of women of all sizes measure their entire worth by the numbers on their bathroom scale. The precious time that is being wasted counting calories, and the resources being spent on useless dieting regimens could surely be put to far better use for humanity. All women deserve to live with respect and enjoy their lives now, rather than at some point in the distant future "when I'm thin enough." Helping professionals are in a key position to incorporate the message of positive self-esteem for all women, regardless of size, into their practice and create meaningful change. It is not enough that we decry the media obsession with thinness. It is up to us to make the world a safer place for fat women to live in peace and good health.

This article addresses three major points. Sport and movement are fundamental to my improved health and well-being, and will be the focus of the first section. Combining feminism, wellness and sport psychology principles and practices allowed me to return from the abyss of depression to the land of the living. These experiences also enabled me to fulfill a lifelong dream, publishing my first book, *Great Shape: The First Exercise Guide for Large Women* (Arbor House/William Morrow, 1988; co-author, Debby Burgard) which I will summarize in the second section. Finally, I will discuss the issue of isolation—a killer disease for fat women—and suggest ways to overcome it en route to healing.

SPORT, FITNESS AND HEALTH: A JOURNEY IN DISCOVERY

Most women my age did not have the good fortune to grow up playing sports. It took the women's movement in the seventies to bring sport into the mainstream of life for millions of women. But in the fifties, in the Midwest where I grew up, sports were considered normal activities for young girls as well as boys, (although active girls were still called tomboys) and I thank my Mom for making sure that my sister and I had the same opportunities as my brother. I was one of those kids who could always tell what season it was by the sports we were playing—bicycling, swimming, tennis and the wonders of Girl Scout camp in the summer; ice skating and sledding like maniacs in the winter. Although I'd been painfully aware of the idea that "fat is ugly" since I was about five or six, it never limited my love for or my participation in sport.

It wasn't until I was in my early teens that being fat began to totally dominate my identity. I stopped ice skating when whether boys asked you to skate or not became more important than trying the jumps and turns I'd always loved. Fat girls were not in great demand as skating partners. By the time I was fifteen, I stopped playing sports altogether because I'd become so self-conscious about being fat (there were no other fat kids on the tennis team, after all). Besides, watching boys play basketball and football was what the other girls were doing, anyway. Girls' P.E. class consisted almost exclusively of calisthenics; exercise had become punishment, boring and lifeless. I was transformed from a joyful sport participant to a passive spectator in a few short years. I began dieting and living from the chin up to desperately try to escape the reality of my fat body. For the next fifteen years, with the exception of a couple of winters spent downhill skiing, I was an experienced and willing couch potato. I know how much my body, my confidence and my spirits suffered from this transformation.

In my early thirties, determined to feel better, I returned to my childhood love of sports and began playing tennis every day. I discovered the field of sport psychology and began learning techniques to relax, concentrate and not allow self-doubt and critical judgements to interfere with my ability to play my best. Playing tennis again, after all the intervening years, was like coming home, and I loved it. I realize now how fortunate I was to have learned movement fundamentals as a child so that I could simply walk out on a court and pick up where I'd left off. Many women never learn the fundamentals as children and must start from scratch as adults. I read everything I could get my hands on about nutrition, fitness, sport psychology, stress management and holistic health. I tried yoga, T'ai Chi and massage. My confidence to try new things was reinforced by my growing competence on the tennis court.

Most importantly, perhaps, I studied feminism and women's health which not only increased my self-respect but opened my eyes to the fact that virtually every woman learns to hate her body regardless of her size. I also began to learn how hard it is to free oneself from oppression. But at least I knew it was important to try, and that I was not alone. Other women were struggling right along with me. It was at that point that I decided I'd waste no further time talking about diets or bemoaning the size of my thighs; women had far more important issues to discuss.

Inspired by all these new ideas, I became a test subject in my own self-help laboratory. I'd been a nurse for many years, but knew mostly about illness. Now, I was learning what becoming healthy and whole was really about. I was fortunate to get a job developing community education and health promotion in an American Indian health project, which was the perfect opportunity to practice professionally what I was learning personally. Little did I know how much I'd learn in the next five years.

In working with Indian people I saw more clearly the insidious and devastating undermining of health that is the result of oppression in America—dire poverty, unemployment, lack of access to health care to name just a few. I learned that regardless of whether oppression is based upon race, gender, economics, body size, or a combination of all of these factors, it creates internalized feelings of shame and self-hatred, as well as conditions and behaviors which are a direct threat to health and well-being. Multiple factors of oppression multiply the problems. But I also saw that problems could be overcome, as Indian women pushed aside multiple barriers that would have stopped me cold. I came to love and respect their courage and tenacity. Many of these women happened to be very large women, and they certainly didn't wait around for the world to give them respect. They respected themselves and got straight on to the business of building a stronger, healthier community. It was the first time I'd had large women as heroes, and they were something.

As my work proceeded it became apparent that empowering people to take care of themselves and prevent disease—through strong cultural identity and self-esteem, and improved nutrition, exercise, stress management practices and social support networks—was fundamental to creating a positive state of health. While access to medical care and health insurance is vital to deal with illness, preventing illness and learning self-care methods are of equal importance. Each of us is our own most powerful resource. While surely we can respect and utilize or in some instances even require the expertise of health care providers to help us, we must also actively work to heal ourselves.

Soon after I began working in my new job I also began running, which became the love of my life for the next six years. I began eating healthier foods and quit my twenty-year cigarette habit. Running gave me both the fitness and the self-confidence to learn softball, cross-country skiing and backpacking. But you know what? I was still fat. Despite all my activity and positive nutritional changes, and although I felt great and was somewhat leaner than when I'd started, at 5'8" 200 pounds and 35% body fat I was still considered "obese" by medical types. My "ideal" weight never materialized.

Lurking in the back of my mind was the nagging thought that while I might be fit and healthy maybe I'd never be thin. Although I'd stopped hating my body, hadn't dieted in more than four years and had thrown away my scales, I still wasn't ready to give up my thin dream. Years and years of believing what the world told me — that it was my fault that I was fat, that being fat was shameful, that I could be thin if I just tried hard enough, and that I could never really be happy until I was thin — made it extremely difficult to let go of the lure of thinness because it felt like giving up the possibility of happiness forever. Besides, I'm stubborn. And I wanted to be thin, dammit! I decided I would just have to try harder and that somehow I was still unconsciously blocking my "thin self" (you know, the one that lives inside every fat person screaming to be free) from emerging. I decided that maybe if I went to graduate school in psychology I could find the answer. As luck would have it, I did. But it was not the answer I thought I'd find.

I entered graduate school determined to link the principles of wellness, feminism and sport psychology and bring this knowledge to women who'd been deprived of enjoying sport and movement. Deprivation of movement is a fundamental disenfranchisement from the body; because of sexism women had not only been objectified but had been denied full access to sport. No wonder it was so hard for us to learn to love our bodies. I also knew from my own experience the power of movement to heal. Through sport psychology I'd learned to appreciate my body from the inside out, giving me tremendous confidence and peace; I wanted to share this learning with women who'd been intimidated by standard sport/exercise environments.

By the time I was ready to write my master's thesis I realized my waiting for the impossible dream of thinness was over. I'd finally had time to delve into the research on dieting, fasting and weight loss surgery more completely, and found the high risk and abysmal failure of these so called "treatments." Books like the *Dieter's Dilemma* (Bennett & Gurin, 1982) finally convinced me that to be fat was not a shameful sin. The health risks of being fat had been exaggerated. Being hated and ridiculed publicly, deprived of employment, education and health insurance, and blamed for a condition that was predicated more upon genetics than personal behavior was the result of social oppression, not scientific fact. And the social oppression of fat people was creating more health problems than any amount of weight ever could. In workshops on unlearning racism and oppression I applied the same principles to unlearning my fat-hating attitudes. I attended performances by Fat Lip Readers' Theater, strongly feminist women in the San Francisco Bay area who use the word "fat" matter-of-factly and with respect, declare fat pride, and ridicule society's obsession with thinness with great wit and style. Where had these women been all my life?

Finally, I'd found my answer. I, Pat Lyons, a fat woman, could live my life in peace. I could be healthy and fit, but I'd always be fat. And being fat was finally O.K. I had a right to respect the body I was born to have, and no one had a right to ridicule or humiliate me any more. Most of all I didn't have the right to ridicule or humiliate myself. It wasn't becoming thin that would make me happy, but learning to accept and love myself could. What a relief! It was like being let out of a dank prison into the full sunshine of the day. Now I could get on with fulfilling my dreams.

After graduate school I began working on our book. It's funny. All my life I thought I'd have to become thin to have my dreams come true. Now, my long time dream of being a published author is a reality. Ironically, if I'd become thin it never would have happened!

GREAT SHAPE: THE FIRST EXERCISE GUIDE FOR LARGE WOMEN

Envision a room filled with happy, healthy dancing women. They twirl and swirl, stretch with catlike grace, and then . . . they get down, honey, and boogie to the beat . . . After dancing themselves into a drenching sweat of pleasure, they cool down, slow down, relax, feel the flush in their cheeks, and luxuriate in the warmth of their bodies. This feels go-o-o-o-d, deep down . . . Now envision that all these healthy women weigh over two hundred pounds . . . did you say "Hot damn? It's about time?"

Great Shape is based on the idea that fat and fit are not mutually exclusive terms. It brings the reality of fitness to women who are tired of the endless cycle of dieting, exercising, quitting and self-badgering in an effort to win acceptance in our size-seven world. Body size is not the determining factor for enjoyment of movement; all women, regardless of size, deserve respectful encouragement, sound information and support to be as healthy and fit as they can be. Debby Burgard and I believe that the pleasures, benefits, challenges and full-out exuberant fun of dance, sport and movement are the birthrights of all people, not just the already athletic and fit. As teenagers, many of us waited in vain to be chosen for teams or as dance partners. Now as adults, we can do the choosing, and can learn to enjoy, not dread, activity.

Regardless of standard exercise propaganda, the purpose of exercise is not to lose weight, but to play and enjoy physical activity for its own sake, as an end in itself. Sport and dance are ways to nourish our bodies, not reduce them, a way to enjoy, empower, and express ourselves more fully. Large women deserve the self-confidence and pleasure of having responsive, capable bodies and good feelings about our physical selves. We need not be ashamed of our fat bodies any longer.

Many large women have finally come to the conclusion that picking a number on the scale and postponing our lives until we reach that number is never going to work. What we really want is a good life, full of friends, enjoyment, and self-respect. To eat what we want when we feel hungry, stop when we're full, move when we feel sluggish, tense, or in need of a lift or some fun, and stop when we're refreshed — then see what our body size is and make peace with it — is a way of living that feels good. And we can have it — now and forever. It is a good life that is *possible*.

But it takes courage to challenge a world that believes we should get thin or get lost. Large women have been treated shabbily by the "no pain, no gain" exercise establishment. By not creating safe activities and environments that welcome rather than ridicule large bodies, exercise enthusiasts who mistakenly equate *thinness* with *fitness* have made the 30 million women in America who wear over a size 16 into objects of scorn. It is, in fact, public ridicule and fear of humiliation that we believe keeps more fat women on the sidelines than any other factor. And it's time women stop being victimized by these attitudes.

Great Shape presents a new way to begin exercise by visualizing what one's exercise preferences might be, looking at what has stopped past efforts, learning how to overcome these obstacles, and finally, finding ways to get a program started that will last. We cover the confusing and controversial research on exercise and weight, specific safety issues, and the more practical aspects of buying shoes, finding large size exercise clothing, choosing a class or activity, the importance of warming up, stretching and cooling down, and what to do about any insults that may come our way. Chapters cover toning and stretching exercises, walking, swimming and other sports, and tips on concentration and body awareness from the field of sport psychology.

The appendix of *Great Shape* features an annotated bibliography, listings of classes and clothing suppliers across the country, and a special section for exercise instructors interested in teaching large women. Finally, opportunities to obtain on-going support, in the form of magazines (*Radiance: The Magazine for Large Women*, published in Oakland, CA) or organizations (Ample Opportunity, Portland, OR; National Association to Aid Fat Americans, chapters nationwide) are also included.

One of the most exciting aspects of *Great Shape* are the photographs of large women swimming, dancing, hiking, bicycling, doing martial arts and playing softball. A picture is worth a thousand words, and photographer Irene Young brought our vision to life. But incredible as it may seem, we had to fight tooth and nail with the publisher to include pictures of active large women — in this, a book about activity for large women! The idea of printing a photograph of a large woman without the word BEFORE underneath it apparently seemed far too risky. But after much struggle, we prevailed. The photographs are living proof that with respect and opportunity, large women can enjoy diverse activities.

Although there are definite safety factors to keep in mind, factors that apply to all new exercisers of any size — learning to monitor one's heart rate, going slowly at first, learning to listen to the messages from our body to avoid injury — virtually any woman can become more active if she chooses. This does not mean exercise is a duty of fat people. We have no more obligation to exercise than anyone else. But neither the world's prejudice nor our own should keep us from an active life.

In *Great Shape*, we emphasize the spirit of recess and play. Exercise has unnecessarily been far too dominated by a work-work-work-out ethic. We invite women to join us and to have fun. Together, whether in dance classes or group hikes, we can also overcome our isolation.

OVERCOMING ISOLATION

If I had a dollar for every hour I spent during my twenties and early thirties at home, watching television and crying into my popcorn because I was so lonely, I'd probably never have to work again. The social prejudice against fat people creates an environment where isolation for protection is understandable and all too common. Social prejudice is also a source of great stress, and the relationship between stress and the development of various illnesses has been extensively discussed in serious medical literature. What is not as well known is that people who experience life's stresses in isolation are at greater risk for both physical and mental health problems (Nuckolls, Cassell, & Kaplan, 1972). One could legitimately argue that the source of problems commonly associated with fatness is not the result primarily of weight, but is instead the result of lives spent painfully alone.

A comprehensive research study conducted with 7,000 residents of Alameda County, California, on the health benefits of social support showed that people with few relationships with other people had death rates that were two to five times higher than those with more supportive social ties. These mortality differences existed independent of standardly defined risk factors such as smoking, drinking and obesity, psychological variables, utilization of health care services and across differences in race, sex and economics

(Berkman & Syme, 1979). In *The Broken Heart: The Medical Consequences of Loneliness*, James Lynch (1977) addresses cardiovascular disease (the most common threat of dire consequences used by physicians to scare people into trying to lose weight) and advances the idea that "even the most elementary forms of human interactions could profoundly influence the heart . . . that medical science had focused all their attention on strictly physical factors—high blood pressure, cigarette smoking, weight, exercise, cholesterol levels, etc.—while completely ignoring the critical importance of human relationships" (Lynch, 1977). It is clear that helping fat people overcome isolation might be the best medicine available to improve our health.

But it is more difficult to overcome isolation than to simply say: "Get out there and make friends!" Fat people have learned that we are supposed to be invisible (a contradiction in terms when you think about it) wear dark clothes, and sit in the back of the room so as not to draw attention to ourselves. We have also learned to avoid each other. Stop and think about the last time you saw a group of six women over two hundred pounds out in public together. It's pretty rare, right? The idea of getting together with other large women outside the context of "curing ourselves" through weight loss may be completely foreign.

Self-help groups, which operate from the assumption that it is easier to reach out to others who share a common experience, can be problematic when the common experiences have a basis in social stigma. The stigmatized may not wish to share one another's company. Many fat women have no other fat friends; many would refuse to consider dating a fat person. We look at a woman fatter than ourselves and breathe a sigh of relief that we are "not as fat as she is." We distance ourselves from women larger than ourselves because we are overwhelmed by fear that we may become like them, that fat is "catching," and staunchly refuse to acknowledge any similarities we may share. This makes all of our lives more difficult than they would be if we were able to willingly reach out to one another. Together we have the power to heal ourselves.

Fat women must create situations where we can come together to share information and support because no one else will do it for us. I'm not talking about Weight Watchers or Overeaters Anonymous, which stigmatize fat and put a premium on food intake and weight loss. I believe we must stop talking about food and weight loss and turn our attention to sharpening our information base, stop mindlessly repeating misinformation like "calories in equals calories out" and cheering each other for losing one quarter of a pound. Our weight is not the issue. Our attitude toward our weight is what holds the key. We must learn what it is we hold dear, what dreams we have put on hold, how to gain the skills and the confidence to attain these goals and how we can learn to better relate to each other despite our misgivings and our fear.

Sport and exercise have been fundamental in helping me learn to love my body, but even after many years of activity I still thought I should be able to become thin. It wasn't until I came together with other fat women to examine the research, discuss serious issues of oppression and, most importantly to play and enjoy ourselves that I finally felt healing occur at the deepest levels of my being. I allowed myself to cry tears of relief and self-acceptance. Finally I was able to love myself.

Every Saturday morning I rush to a large-women-only swim, where women my size and much larger shed the fear of criticism and frolic in the comfort of warm water. Many swim laps; others play volley ball; everyone enjoys each other's company. To see all of us together, in a full array of gorgeous, colorful swim suits made by one of the swim organizers, has changed my life. When working with American Indians, I had the first experience of being with many other fat people and not having it make any difference in terms of respect and human caring. At the swim I get the same feeling. It is a profoundly healing experience. And I am proud of all of us.

No one is meant to live from the chin up. It deprives us of living as fully integrated human beings. Learning that our bodies can move with grace and power at any size, can bring us pleasure as we gradually unlearn the lies the world has embedded in our psyches — that our bodies are ugly, clumsy and should remain hidden. Our body is our anchor to the moment. With each breath we can tune into our inner strength. Our body does not lie or give us rationalizations. If given half a chance it can simply be our home, warm and cozy, whether we're actually at home or out in the world.

Together, women can help create a world where each of us lives with respect in our body whatever our size. It is a goal that deserves our full attention.

REFERENCES

Bennett, W., & Gurin, J. (1982). *The Dieter's Dilemma*. New York: Basic Books.

Berkman, L., & Syme, S. (1979). Social Networks, Host Resistance and Mortality: A Nine-Year Follow-up Study of Alameda County Residents. *American Journal of Epidemiology, 109*, 186-204.

Lynch, J. (1977). *The Broken Heart: The Medical Consequences of Loneliness*. New York: Basic Books.

Nuckolls, K.B., et al. (1972). Psychosocial Assets, Life Crises and the Prognosis of Pregnancy. *American Journal of Epidemiology, 95*.

Ample Opportunity for Fat Women

Nancy Barron
Barbara Hollingsworth Lear

SUMMARY. Ample Opportunity provides social support for body acceptance. The organization sponsors physical activities, workshops, and information-sharing which promote physical and mental health for fat women. Ample Opportunity acknowledges the social stigma associated with fatness in this culture and creates positive action toward social change. The philosophy, practices, and organizational model are described. There is opportunity for coalition building among fat women, health and mental health professionals, and organizations like Ample Opportunity which support a positive lifestyle not dependent on weight reduction. The philosophy and principles of Ample Opportunity are relevant to psychotherapy, and specific applications useful to therapists are developed.

INTRODUCTION

The Ample Opportunity (AO) organization works to assure accessibility to a high quality of life for fat women and to create a social environment more accepting of all body sizes. The organization emphasizes self-esteem, positive experiences for personal growth, mutual support, social action, information, and satisfying physical activity. We stress the wisdom of our experience as well as the knowledge gained from empirical findings.

This article will consider the stigma and fear of fatness, the phi-

Nancy Barron, PhD (Psychology), Ample Opportunity, 5370 NW Roanoke, Portland, OR 97229, coordinates Multnomah County emergency mental health services and manages Ample Opportunity. She develops and facilitates many of the AO workshops. Teaching bellydancing for emotional growth is the most fun.

Barbara Hollingsworth Lear, Ample Opportunity, 5370 NW Roanoke, Portland, OR 97229, is a student of anthropology and a founder of Ample Opportunity. She is currently researching the changing role of women in American rodeo.

losophy and organization of AO, and the relationship of these to therapeutic intervention. AO is relevant to therapists in many ways. Where organized activities are available, they are a useful referral source. Where not, the philosophy, principles and information can be an aid to therapists and clients who are concerned with issues of fatness.

Our culture strongly stigmatizes fatness. For instance, the media, with rare exception, tout only young, thin women and generally depict fat women as humorous, villainous, or maternal. The stigma affects the social reality and occupational potential of fat women. For example, one sample of human service professionals reacted significantly less positively toward a young woman interested in entering the field who appeared fat than toward the same woman who appeared slender (Benson, Severs, Tatgenhorst, & Loddengaard, 1980). A sample of mental health therapists rated the description of a prospective client as more severely disturbed if she looked fat in a picture than if she did not (Young & Powell, 1985).

Most women of all sizes internalize this negative social evaluation of fatness. They find their bodies unacceptably fat and fear that others do also (e.g., Dyrenforth, Wooley, & Wooley, 1980).

The social stigma is supported by a notion of fatness as unhealthy. Although the psychological burden is the greatest health risk (Wadden & Stunkard, 1985), methods of treating obesity consider fatness a disease and fat women as patients to comply with physical regimens (Consensus Development Conference, 1985). Perhaps fatness should not be treated at all (Wooley & Wooley, 1984). A recent review of research findings suggests that health risks are minimal or not causally related to fatness and that fatness also has some health benefits (Ernsberger & Haskew, 1987), so health is probably not the central issue. People with chronic diseases do not face the same negative prejudice as fat people. Many barriers to societal rewards do exist, and fatness, often considered the "fault" of the individual, is used as a means of rationalizing discriminatory practices.

We in AO believe that all members of society will benefit from greater size acceptance, that fat phobia is largely an issue of social control of women, and that fat women need not lose weight in order to live a healthy, full life. We believe that many persons in the helping professions can exert positive influence toward size acceptance and more positive attitudes toward fat women.

This article presents four years' experience with the AO program and philosophy. We offer information on activities, practices, and issues and discuss the role of therapists in developing ample opportunity for fat women.

DESCRIPTION OF THE
AMPLE OPPORTUNITY PROGRAM

Roots

Ample Opportunity grew out of consciousness raising groups of the women's movement, the self-help group tradition, the wellness movement, and the experiences of the authors as fat women, social scientists, and professionals (Barron, Eakins, & Wollert, 1984). AO, created for the self-defined benefit of the participants, is a response to a perceived need for experiences which validate our realities and create an environment in which participants can maximize their individual potential and quality of life. We stress self-acceptance and encouragement to live now, not wait until we are thinner.

Organization

The authors began the organization in 1984 in a west coast metropolitan area of approximately a million persons. An advisory council of fat women gave program input and volunteer support. The advisory council was disbanded in 1985, but volunteers still staff all activities. An unpaid volunteer coordinator keeps the organization functioning in an integrated way. A core of volunteers who are also participants in AO help generate organizational activities. The organization is heir to the problems of volunteer organizations such as recruitment and training of new volunteers, difficulties in communication among the many persons involved and lack of follow-through due to other demands on the volunteers from, for example, paid work and family.

The senior author facilitates many of the activities. Additional facilitators, recruited both locally and nationally, may receive honoraria; the volunteer staff receives organizational benefits. The moderately-priced activities are partially supported by users' fees, and work exchange is often available. AO is non-profit. A board is currently being constituted to provide policy refinement, develop resources, and obtain federal tax exempt status as a non-profit organization.

Participants

The women in AO range from young adolescents to women in their seventies; the modal age is approximately 35. Occupational status ranges from unemployed, including some who receive disability benefits, through middle class professionals, business women, students, and homemakers. While no one grouping seems typical, the upper middle class is underrepresented. Reflective of the metropolitan population, most women are white, heterosexual, and married. The women are very diverse in both politics and lifestyle. Our clinical impression is that the members' mental health does not differ from that of the general population. Most women in AO are substantially fat, i.e., have a body mass index above 30. The range of fatness in AO varies from about 15-150% over the average weight of the general population. Some women of average weight have recently chosen to join in on some of the activities.

Program

Activities offered have varied depending on demand and the interest of the core volunteers and the co-authors. Early programs included fat awareness gatherings, folk dance, yoga, T'ai Chi, and volleyball. Participants developed a resource guide to goods and services for fat women in the metropolitan area. Later programs included support groups, community education, outdoor activities such as rafting and canoe trips, hot springs expeditions, and community education. From the start, there have been swims, bellydance, the monthly newsletter, growth-oriented workshops, and a semi-annual large-size clothing exchange. Some of these activities are described here in order to illustrate more fully the nature of participation in AO.

Fat Awareness Gatherings. Women of all sizes gathered to increase their awareness of issues of fatness. First, each woman shared a brief history and current issues of her life concerning fatness. This sharing quickly built a feeling of cohesion in the group. Then the facilitators briefly summarized frequently-held misconceptions about fatness and current research findings. The focus shifted then to personal experience of fatness. Small group discussions formed around issues identified in the initial sharing. The philosophy, program, and upcoming activities of Ample Opportunity were described, and the group closed by sharing positive affirmations.

Workshops. Workshops have addressed fatness and depression, sexuality, shame, self-love, personal journaling, physical activity, and body image. One workshop is held each month except when supplanted by outdoor activities during the summer. Workshops have been given in other states at conferences or for preexisting groups.

As an example, "From Shame to Self-Love" began with an introduction which framed shame as a universal developed experience and a special dynamic for women who are fat. The women shared experiences in which they had felt shamed. We reviewed the clinical knowledge of shame, information about fatness, then looked at how fatness is shamed. We created a repertoire of coping strategies with which to counter the shaming experiences. Finally, we focused on the principles and practices of self-loving.

Swims. The twice-weekly drop-in swim hour is for substantially fat women. A volunteer hostess greets and orients new swimmers, takes the swimming fee, and acts as liaison with the woman lifeguard of the rented city pool. As volunteer talent is available, water aerobics are offered. Pool space is divided to accommodate lap swimmers, women improving their strokes, aerobic exercisers, and those who want to bob quietly and chat.

Bellydance for Emotional Growth. Bellydance is presented as an ancient women's art suited for bodies of ample proportions. AO offers ongoing six-week bellydance workshops in which fat women support one another's enjoyment and emotional growth, become more aware of and comfortable with their bodies, increase strength, suppleness and aerobic fitness, explore the tradition of women bellydancing, and gain skill. Each woman is encouraged to improvise her own dancing garb, which ranges from sweatsuits to full Middle Eastern costume. Each week we check in with one another as we arrive, dance together what we learned the week before, share with one another the thoughts and feelings that come up, and add new dance experience.

Newsletter. *Ample Information* (Barron & Lear, 1988) is now entering its fifth volume. Most subscriptions are local, but an increasing number are scattered across the nation. The format includes articles, AO news and plans, an explanation of some portion of AO philosophy, a calendar of the next month's activities, and art depicting active fat women in a positive light. The articles are generally written by AO women, although several other professionals have contributed articles in their areas of expertise.

The feature article may be a first-person account of living as a fat woman, a summary of recent research or a relevant new book, or an essay on personal growth. Representative articles have included: a review of the 1985 NIH Consensus Development Conference; measures of body image; holiday sanity for fat women; feminist therapy; the high visibility of fatness; insights into fatness that come with losing weight; lifespan issues of fatness; health and exercise; research and prejudice; comparisons and self-worth; sexuality; fat oppression as a form of violence against women; aspertame; and notes of a fat therapist.

Community Education. The partners and volunteers provide training for such groups as battered women, high school and college classes, school mental health programs, and naturopathic college students. A graduate/undergraduate university psychology class has been developed by the senior author focused on self-image and body size. The county health promotion section has procured AO worship for its employees.

Practices

AO attempts to base its practices on its values. Several relevant practices are: using the word "fat," offering activities for fat women only, and incorporating feminist principles into the organization.

Using the Word Fat. Popular euphemisms for fat are inaccurate and carry connotations which deprecate fat women. Obese is a medical term based on the premise that fat is disease resulting from eating too much; "large" hides fat among tall or large-boned. "Overweight" gives undue authority to the insurance charts that imply there is a proper weight which one can be over. We deliberately chose the word fat because it describes us. And, we work for the day when fat will lose its flinch value and be descriptive, not pejorative.

Fat Women Only. Most of the activities AO produces are for fat women only. We are aware that many of the issues which affect fat women are of concern to all women, for example, sexual objectification and discrimination, the tendency to blame ourselves for things not under our control, cultural obsession with body image. Yet, protected space in which fatness is the norm allows women to relax, build skills, and bond with one another around a common concern with fewer invidious comparisons.

Fat Facilitators and the Interpersonal Experience of Moving. In AO activities, we attend to how it feels to be a fat body in motion and attempt to make moving a pleasant, self-enhancing experience. Private, protected space for many of the physical activities avoids the potential for ridicule or embarrassment that we may experience when we exercise in public. In relearning the delights of moving, we choose non-competitive activities which are relatively free of demands for special gear and which an individual can do at any skill level. We provide social support for moving.

Using fat women as facilitators makes physical activity easier for fat women. If we see a body moving in certain ways, and that body is like our own, then it is easier for us to believe that we can learn to move that way than if the body is younger, slimmer, or otherwise unlike our own. This likeness fosters encouragement, confidence, understanding of the activity, and appropriate pacing. We can set more realistic goals; we don't have to translate; our kinesthetic empathy comes more easily.

A Feminist Organization. AO is a feminist organization. Its mission is to benefit women, especially fat women.

Fatness is disproportionally a women's issue. Biologically, women have a larger percent of body fat than men; socially, we face far narrower, more prescriptive, more strongly sanctioned norms for fatness. The prejudice and social control are more blatantly directed at women. As members of the group experiencing this prejudice, we have the greatest vested interest in combatting it. According to the AO motto, "A good life is the best revenge."

In AO we strive to improve the status of women by supporting each woman's efforts toward a positive self-concept as a worthwhile individual in her own right. We work with fat women because much of our expertise is generated from living as fat women. Our understanding and empathy can be greater with those most similar to ourselves. Mutual support is built most readily around a common core experience. Especially because of the great diversity of women who approach AO, homogeneity around the core experiences as fat women is important to the ability to bond with each other to our mutual benefit. We also support public education toward size acceptance and women's rights.

Issues

In contrast to the practices above, several controversial areas remain, namely, weight loss, how fat is fat, and the optimum organization.

Weight Loss. Given an inherited, slightly modifiable range of fatness which the body defends and the likelihood that, at the end of each diet we face weight gain in excess of weight lost after dieting because of damaged metabolism (Bennett & Gurin, 1982), AO does not recommend diets. Participants' personal views on diets are accepted, but we encourage self-acceptance and a healthy lifestyle including relaxed eating of good food, moving in ways that are rewarding, and enjoying both social action and sociability with other fat women. AO continues to educate others that fat women can be healthy women and that weight loss is not necessarily evidence of improved health. And, if we can transform the energy women spend worrying about body size into positive social action, the benefit to cultural quality of life could be immense.

How Fat Is Fat? This simple question was the most agonizing dilemma we faced. We have found that we have no clear answer since fatness is gradient, not a dichotomy. Different ranges of fatness are associated with different experiences, and women who are not at all fat also struggle with issues of fatness. Despite AO's attempt to leave fatness self-defined, early in the life of the organization, many of the very fat women on the advisory council felt strongly that only very fat women should be eligible for membership. They believed that less fat women didn't know the full range of pain and rejection. Less fat women thereby felt betrayed and feared they did not fit either in the mainstream or in the fat group. This polarization, reminiscent of how black is Black and feminist splintering, is another manifestation of internalized prejudice. It is very difficult to settle this issue in a way that protects the *balance* of rights and sensitivities of a broad range of fat women. The issue has not been settled; guidelines are again elastic, and we rely largely on self-definition.

The Optimum Organization. Barriers to recruitment, financial issues, and growth influence organizational viability. Since AO is small and self-supporting, free or low-cost publicity is used. There are cost barriers for many participants. Although pricing is minimal and work exchange is available, women have less money than men, and since fatness is somewhat correlated with social class due to selection, discrimination, and nutrition (Haellstrom & Nappa, 1981), fat women have less money yet. Until activities burgeon, hiring staff is not possible, and, without staff time to fully develop programs and maximize opportunities to get the information out, it is difficult to recruit. Specially-targeted activities also depend on staff expansion. Resource development is difficult because human service funding channels do not identify the AO mission as fundable because they are still focused on thinner women, not happier, healthier women.

There are also conceptual barriers. The AO philosophy is unfamiliar, counter to the popular media, and often misunderstood. Some women believe that they will be fine when they lose weight and that joining AO would be "giving up," admitting "failure." Others have retreated from the discrimination into isolation; involvement for them is frightening and difficult. Some have difficulty with the diversity of lifestyles represented by the members or with AO's feminist orientation. Our program attempts to address these barriers by increasing awareness, fostering conscious inclusiveness, and bridging.

THE THERAPIST AND AMPLE OPPORTUNITY
FOR FAT WOMEN

The AO principles and philosophy can be generalized from fat women helping one another to therapists working with fat women. Reciprocal communication between AO and therapists has been a priority. Referral is one active mechanism for communication. Although most members are self-referred, some are referred to AO by therapists as an exercise opportunity, some for support, some for political relevance, some to integrate personal gains in a positive social context. AO also refers women for concentrated personal work to therapists who evidence maximum size acceptance. Although many fat women are healthy and eat well, some do suffer from eating disorders. Some suffer from poor physical or mental health. Some also suffer from encounters with medical personnel who focus on fat as the cause of unrelated injuries or illnesses. These women benefit from treatment as well as involvement in AO. AO and psychotherapy can be complementary, often creating a positive synergy for both client and therapist. When therapists' philosophies are counter to AO, there may also be a dynamic tension.

AO provides a range of professional training. Some women are both AO members and practicing professionals, many in health or mental health services. Some facilitate special AO activities in their areas of expertise or write articles for our newsletter. AO facilitators sometimes consult with professionals not in AO who care about safe, beneficial movement and a positive experience for fat women. We encourage professionals to become knowledgeable and to support size acceptance.

AO draws heavily on the empirical knowledge base concerning the etiology, social stigma, and modifiability of fatness. The "problem" is not fatness, the problem is the negative social context which is based on a set of popular beliefs that are unsubstantiated or overestimated. For example:

Popular Belief	Empirical Information
Fattness represents gluttony or an eating disorder.	Fat people cannot consistently be demonstrated to eat more or differently than thin people (Kissileff, Jordan, & Levitz, 1978).

Fatness represents ill health.	Such evidence is weak, correlational, and specific to a few disorders; also fatness is associated with health benefits (Ernsberger & Hasket, 1987).
Diet and exercise will make a fat woman acceptably thin.	Good eating and exercising influences health and fitness more than weight (Krotkiewski, Mandroukas, Sjostrom, Sullivan, Wettergvist & Bjorntorp, 1979, Folkens & Sime, 1981, Lyons & Burgard, 1988, Moore & Leklem, 1988).
Dieting will make a fat person thin forever	Cycles of weight loss and weight gain through dieting change the metabolism so that lost weight is gained despite average or restrained eating (Bennett & Gurin, 1982).
Fatness is readily changed if one chooses	The heritability of fatness is demonstrated in the relationship between body/mass of biological but not adopted parents and their children, especially mothers and daughters (Stunkard et al., 1986).

We encourage therapists to consider critically personal beliefs about fatness, to become familiar with recent research such as the studies above, and to come to peace with personal issues around fatness, which, left unexamined, are almost inevitably prejudicial in our culture. As part of this consideration, the therapist can inform herself of organizations or activities similar to AO which exist in her community, refer clients, volunteer her expertise, and make known her principle of size acceptance.

Often there is nothing in the community similar to AO. In that case, the therapist can help create opportunities. Some practices of AO can be incorporated into any therapeutic intervention involving fat women. For instance, a therapist may suggest as a worthy treatment goal acceptance of oneself as a fat woman. Perhaps she may introduce the use of the word fat as a non-judgmental term and assist a client to take the negative connotations out of it. She may suggest "homework" for a client involving becoming at home in her body and explore with her the attendant barriers and satisfactions. She may wish to share some of her personal journey around issues of self-acceptance.

As fat women, we need therapists who hear our experience without presuming that they know it better or that our eating or our psyches are disordered just because we are fat. We need therapists well-informed on current information about fatness who do not succumb to popular but inaccurate beliefs and who may help us refute some of those same beliefs. Therapists can understand that we daily interact with a hostile social environment in which those most likely to challenge us on the basis of our fatness are those closest to us. Fat women deserve assistance toward health and mental health gains unrelated to our fatness. We need support in becoming more aware, more self-accepting and gentle with ourselves, and more assertive in trying to influence people toward size acceptance.

Left largely unaddressed are the complex relationships among mental health system attitudes toward fatness, effects of psychotropic medications (with side effects of weight gain), the influence of socioeconomic and gender status, and diagnosis and treatment planning for fat women not focused on weight loss. Informed, aware therapists are more likely to prescribe treatment which is congruent with knowledge of the dynamics of fatness and understanding of the phenomenology of fat women. The mental health system can also promote health for fat women by assuring opportunities for training for administrators, staff, and clients around issues of fatness.

Many aspects of program evaluation and research deserve attention in the future. During the last four years, AO has struggled to communicate a perspective distilled from the experience of fat women and recent research. The recent popularity of the term "size acceptance" is an indicator that social change is occurring, although the link between the action and the effect is putative.

The efficacy of AO is indicated by its survival, the personal experience of members and their associates, and glimmers of change in social attitudes. The organizational goals provide a substantial list of outcomes deserving of investigation. We need research which asks questions based on informed size acceptance rather than prejudicial assumptions and which uses rigorous, inventive, quasi-experimental design characterized by minimally intrusive measures. Funding for research focused on the quality of life of fat women is difficult to find. One grant proposal resulted in being offered consultation on constructing a randomly assigned, controlled treatment study of weight loss—hardly what we had in mind.

CONCLUSION

Women experience multiple benefits from the philosophy and activities of Ample Opportunity which address coping with the negative social context of fatness. Unfortunately, this sort of organization is unavailable in most areas. However, therapists interacting with fat women can enhance their therapeutic effect by incorporating AO principles into their practice. Information, self-awareness, empathy, and behavior congruent with size acceptance will strengthen the potential benefit a therapist may help create for fat women.

REFERENCES

Barron, N., Eakins, L. I., & Wollert, R. W. (1984) Fat group: A SNAP-launched self-help group for overweight women. *Human Organization, 43*, 44-49.

Barron, N., & Lear, B. (Eds.) (1985, 1986, 1987, 1988) *Ample Information Newsletter, 1, 2, 3, 4.* Ample Opportunity, 5370 NW Roanoke Ln., Portland, OR, 97229. $12/year, 11 issues.

Bennett, W., & Gurin, J. (1982) *The dieter's dilemma: The scientific case against dieting as a means of weight control.* New York: Basic Books, Inc.

Benson, P. L., Severs, D., Tatgenhorst, J, & Loddengaard, N. (1980) The social costs of obesity: A non-reactive field study. *Social Behavior and Personality, 8*, 91-96.

Consensus Development Conference. (1985) Health implications of obesity. *Annals of Internal Medicine, 103*, 1073-1077.

Dyrenforth, S. R., Wooley, O. W., & Wooley, S. C. (1980) A woman's body in a man's world: A review of findings on body image and weight control. In J. R. Kaplan (Ed.), *A woman's conflict: The special relationship between women and food.* Englewood Cliffs, N.J.: Prentice-Hall, Inc.

Ernsberger, P., & Haskew, P. (1987) Rethinking obesity. *Journal of Obesity and Weight Regulation, 6*, 58-137.

Folkens, C. H., & Sime, W. E. (1981) Physical fitness training and mental health. *American Psychologist, 36*, 373-389.

Haellstroem, T., & Noppa, H. (1981) Obesity in women in relation to mental illness, social factors and personality traits. *Journal of Psychosomatic Research, 25,* 75-82.

Kissilef, K. S., Jordan, H. A., & Levitz, L. S. (1978) Eating habits of obese and normal weight humans. *International Journal of Obesity, 2,* 379.

Krotkiewski, M., Mandroukas, K., Sjostrom, L., Sullivan, L., Wetterqvist, H., & Bjorntorp, P. (1979) Effects of long term physical training on body fat, metabolism, and blood pressure in obesity. *Metabolism, 28,* 650-658.

Lyons, P., & Burgard, D. (1988) *Great shape: The first exercise guide for large women.* New York: Arbor House.

Moore, J., & Leklem, J. (1988) Paper read at the Annual Meeting of the Federation of American Societies for Experimental Biology.

Stunkard, A. J., Sorensen, T. I. A., Hanis, C., Teasdale, T. W., Chakraborty, R., Schull, W. J., & Schulsinger, F. (1986) An adoption study of human obesity. *The New England Journal of Medicine, 314*(4), 193-198.

Wadden, T. A., & Stunkard, A. J. (1985) Social and psychological consequences of obesity. *Annals of Internal Medicine, 103,* 1050-1051.

Wooley, S., & Wooley, O. (1984) Should obesity be treated at all? In A. J. Stunkard and E. Steller (Eds.), *Eating and its disorders.* New York: Raven Press.

Young, L. M., & Powell, B. (1985) The effects of obesity on the clinical judgements of mental health professionals. *Journal of Health and Social Behavior, 26,* 233-246.

Fat Is Generous, Nurturing, Warm . . .

Angela Barron McBride

SUMMARY. Three years of journal entries are analyzed as a means of understanding the experience of one fat woman. One revelation was the extent to which thoughts and feelings were organized around the root metaphors of "bigger is better" and "more is better." Being large is associated with being exceptional, expansive, strong, warm, generous, nurturing. These *positive* connections are regarded as important to recognize in a world that regards being "overweight" as necessarily negative. Recognizing the positive associations can have the effect of making sense out of habitual behaviors, and can set the stage for searching for new meanings which are health-enhancing.

Over a three-year period, I kept a journal on my experience as a fat woman. I saw myself as a highly competent person in every area of my life with one exception—I had been fat all my life. I rather whimsically decided that I would be able to lose weight if only I had myself in therapy, so I decided to enter into a dialogue with myself using paper and pen. In this enterprise, I was to be the person with the problem *and* the person seeking to make sense out of the experience. I had firsthand knowledge of what it was like to struggle with the diagnosis of obesity and my training as both a psychiatric nurse and psychologist had prepared me to discern the themes that emerge

Angela Barron McBride is Professor and Associate Dean for Research at Indiana University School of Nursing. She is also Adjunct Professor in the Department of Psychology (Purdue University School of Science at Indianapolis), in the Department of Psychiatry (Indiana University School of Medicine), and in Women's Studies (Indiana University-Purdue University at Indianapolis). She wrote one of the position papers for developing the National Institute of Mental Health's research agenda for women's mental health.

93

once the patterns behind a series of discrete instances of behavior come into focus.

Diaries/journals have historically been a way for women to confront the truth of their lives. Many a teenage girl has used a diary to help her decode her thoughts and feelings. Moffat and Painter (1974, p. 5) described the form as an important outlet for women "partly because it is an analogue to their lives" in the sense of being emotional, fragmentary, interrupted, private, daily, formless, and as endless as their tasks. The form provides a means to overthrow artificial divisions between subjective and objective through critical self-reflection (Keller, 1982). It is a form which lends itself to consciousness raising:

> Taking situated feelings and common detail (common here meaning both ordinary and shared) as the matter of political analysis, it [consciousness raising] explores the terrain that is most damaged, most contaminated, yet therefore most women's own, most intimately known, most open to reclamation. (MacKinnon, 1982, p. 536)

Diaries/journals are ideally suited to the painstaking task of actively constructing "truth" out of self-understanding.

Anything connected with being fat seemed grist for my journal. Special attention was paid to describing in detail events which engendered a powerful emotional response. The primary focus was always on recognizing what the experiencing individual knows by scrutinizing layer after layer of thoughts and feelings over time. Since losing weight was an issue in my life, there were many passages on the experience of dieting, but there also was corresponding attention paid to the overall experience of someone who is fat. Over time, there was some movement away from being exclusively preoccupied with the negative to admitting positive thoughts and feelings. Most impressions were recorded on the very day that they were experienced. A tape recorder was used as an adjunct to paper and pen because it allowed for a stream-of-consciousness approach: you talk and dart from topic to topic without making connections, and later listen to the tapes only to find that there are connections that can be made. The understandings reached using this technique were then written up as part of that week's entries.

SAMPLE DIARY ENTRIES 1979-1982

What follows are excerpts from the journal which communicate some sense of the issues raised over time:

August 18, 1979

I dislike tiny women. Chihuahua women. For so long, I have wanted to be seen as competent, strong, generous, solid. I automatically label women who are slender, gorgeous and frail as useless — yapping dogs to be petted.

September 1, 1979

A diet is not the stuff of Shakespearean tragedy, but I feel like a female Lear lunging around and around. I am pompous, foolish, lost, blind to everything but appetites that are babyish at core. I feel enraged because I have to be careful about what I eat, when I would rather see myself as a person with an immense appetite for life.

September 9, 1979

This weekend I came to appreciate just how much I have ceased to be involved in cooking. Not only has my husband been assuming responsibility for cooking dinner on the three evenings when I get away from work late in the day, but he now plans more and more of the weekend meals, too. Because he is not the prima donna I am in the kitchen, he has managed to involve both daughters in meal preparation more than I ever did. Instead of showing my love for my family with the preparation of some new delicacy, I am reduced (that's how it feels) to accepting their culinary offerings. So much of my ego has been built on compliments that I have garnered as an exceptional cook that I now feel a mere shadow of my former self.

January 2, 1980

In the Polish Catholic community where I grew up, a girl was supposed to have either a figure or brains, but not both. To those who did, people never failed to say something like "And she's smart, too; can you imagine that?" While I have always had some sense that my size protected me from the pitfalls of being a mere sex object, I only realized today the extent to which my size may have actually served the purpose of allowing people to acknowledge my intelligence. Long ago, I may have made some preconscious trade-off: People will think I am "too much" and harass me if I am both attractive and bright, why not put your effort into being bright because that at least is of enduring value?

January 31, 1980

I have been thinking today about Miss Piggy of Muppet Show fame. She is bright, strong, and does not suffer fools easily. Bedecked in lavender satins with her long blonde curls swishing about her, she is my kind of modern woman — one who has a taste both for jewels from admirers and for independence. It is not surprising to me that Miss Piggy is the only female character on the Muppet Show to achieve star status. In many situations, only a substantial woman may be viewed as having substance. Miss Piggy enjoys throwing her weight around, but doesn't she have to have weight even to be noticed and taken seriously?

February 1, 1980

Will I be able to stand my self reduced? Lesser . . . minor . . . abridged . . . diminished . . . dwindling . . . negligible . . . fading . . .

February 10, 1980

All of my life has been devoted to becoming the "big girl" my parents wanted me to be — meaning mature, serious, remarkable, prodigious, extraordinary. I am afraid that my interests will not be widespread if I am not widespread. I do not want to be the weaker sex. Conventional femininity means diminution, invisibility, being lightweight. I rejected those images long ago. *Fat* chance that I'll ever be the *little* woman!

February 15, 1980

I wonder if women's special problem with food did not start with Eve and the apple. Eve wanted "more" out of life, and food became the symbolic representation of her cravings for knowledge. Male scholars like to see apple-eating as a symbol for sexual desire, but Eve's daughters may be closer to the real meaning when they equate food with existential hungerings to be divinities themselves.

February 22, 1980

Many nurses are fat. I think that is because the traditional image of a nurse is one who is strong, maternal, comfortable, and patient. To be well-rounded and pleasant may get construed as involving being round and having soft edges. Traits that are positive may subtly become intertwined in the mind with physical manifestations of those qualities.

March 14, 1980

When I was growing up in east Baltimore, not one woman in my neighborhood looked svelte. I have escaped overstuffed houses and have the veneer of culture I desperately wanted after a steady diet of hillbilly records. I have escaped my childhood, but not quite. My exterior reflects a working class background. I still look as if I am carrying the weight of the world on my shoulders . . . the face and form of a peasant woman. After repudiating my roots so much, I find myself unable to disassociate myself from an outward show of solidarity with my old neighborhood.

May 2, 1980

Cassius had a lean and hungry look, and was tagged as dangerous. I look pillowy; no one looking at me need fear my ambitions when they are encased in fatty inertia. I have them hidden under a surface pliancy.

June 14, 1980

I am not a *femme fatale*. I prefer to be nurturing rather than devastating. No vixen-thin siren drawing men to their doom, I prefer to be Madonna round, and take pride in having chosen to be largehearted, bounteous, hospitable, and indulgent rather than shallow, spindly, vacuous, discontented, and narrowminded.

January 18, 1981

I spy a television commercial that features a male "authority" extolling the benefits to be derived from joining a particular "figure salon." He says, "Girls, you want to keep your New Year's resolution and get back your youthful figure," and I know why I never wanted a youthful figure in the first place. I couldn't handle being someone's "girl." I want to lose weight in order to look and feel better, but certainly not for his sake.

February 17, 1981

Five of us were sitting in the sauna after swimming, and the conversation turned to our own girth. One woman lamented the weight she had gained in the last year, but said she had always liked heavier people — "There is more to them." She patted her belly as you would a lovable but impish child, and smiled. I smiled, too.

October 28, 1981

I want to be able to present my point of view (questioning authority), and have it accorded the respect of a mainstream position. I want to be highly visible, but not stick out. I want to avoid disapproval, but have my position be regarded as substantive. I experience the same dilemma with my physical appearance. I hide under my fatty comforter, but the pillowy look makes me even more visible. I am noticed; I want to be, but I don't want to be.

March 1, 1982

My grandmother regarded big numbers as an accomplishment. Her blood pressure would soar to 210/120 and she would take pride in her score the way a Pac Man addict does. Her disregard was a death-defying trick. She prided herself on rising above mere mortal preoccupations, and so do I.

April 19, 1982

Someone picked me up at an airport and remarked on how lightly I travel. What was meant as a statement of fact, I took as a compliment for traveling unencumbered. I have always looked with disdain on women who cannot negotiate easily because their vanity requires them to travel with clothes for all moods and different creams for different parts of their bodies. I have consolidated all my baggage, so it is just *me*.

BIG IS BETTER

As a person who has always known that she would wish to be thin (meaning able to eat desserts without anyone commenting on my eating habits) if some obliging· genie would offer to meet one heart's desire, I was surprised to see that on the other side of my mortification with being fat is a part of me that regards fat as something very positive. To me, it means being nurturing, warm, lavish, hearty, and a host of other praiseworthy qualities. In a very real sense, to gain is to become gainful (not ungainly).

It was very difficult for me to see through the negative to the positive. Society constantly berates the fat woman for her girth, and the affected individual joins in this cacophony of hateful abuse. It took the hundreds of pages of a three-year journal for me to appreciate fully how much I have wanted to become lean, understated, self-contained, abstemious, and delicate but continue to value highly being effusive, lavish, emotional, unconstrained, and hearty. "Fat" for me does not just conjure up society's negative images, but calls to mind fecundity, prosperity, expansiveness. To be "large" is to be great, substantial, extensive benevolent, strong. "Thin," by contrast, is not necessarily associated in the mind with health; it is also associated with lean times, being insubstantial, shallow, feeble, frail, insufficient.

The journal enabled me to realize the extent to which my world of childhood had been organized around certain root metaphors— "bigger is better" and "more is better." Having a good appetite was something you wanted; it was regarded as a gift from God. Picky eaters were bound to be picky people—not good company in this vale of tears. A good appetite meant that you had a zest for life, gusto. The child who was a good eater could be counted on to do well—get a good job, make a solid marriage, take care of her/his parents in their old age. The thin would, by contrast, put a week's salary into clothes and be too self-centered to bother with you.

Cultures are organized around certain root metaphors that play a role in defining our everyday realities (Lakoff & Johnson, 1980). These linguistic structures serve as a shorthand of sorts for what we take to be self-evident. We are not normally aware of the conceptual system that informs what we pay attention to and how we think, as well as what we actually wind up doing, so confrontation of personal values can be an important step in producing significant behavior change (Schwartz & Inbar-Saban, 1988).

The notion that "bigger is better" leads to all sorts of associations between size and importance. A large person may be viewed as superior, healthy, generous, profound, towering, powerful, remarkable, eminent. On the other hand, every metaphor has the possibility of being turned on its side as values change, especially when the root metaphor no longer seems to correspond with physical experience. Medical reports about the dangers of cholesterol/sugar and television images of famine make "bigger is better" seem dubious as an absolute value, for the phrase has come to be associated with being wasteful, selfish, clumsy, outrageous, gross, sick, immoderate, and out of control by the general public. It should be noted that the validity of those reports has been questioned by Ernsberger and Haskew (1987).

The truth or falsehood of a metaphor is not something that can be subject to debate. Rather, the issue is how a particular metaphor influences us and what actions are sanctioned (consciously and unconsciously) by it. Once we have accepted a metaphor, we focus only on what it highlights; we are less likely to attend to those experiences that might call the metaphor into question. We draw inferences and set goals on the basis of how we structure our experience by means of metaphor.

As a result of the journal, I understand the extent to which weight and food have served a symbolic function in my life. There was some connection in my mind between the A+ and the "pretty plus" dress sizes. Being big protected me from experiencing all the sexual pressures that a slim teenager might have encountered, and for which my parents seemed to be as ill-prepared as I. Hiding under the protection of always looking pregnant was comfortable, serviceable; looking maternal made me look like a caregiver. It was also a way of being rebellious without appearing to be so. The trouble is that some of those connections are dated and dubious given my current problems with hypertension and achy joints.

Once a person has gotten in touch with the unconscious positive connections, the task is not to repudiate the old metaphor (for that is to repudiate yourself), but to start searching for new meanings that seem appropriate for a changing situation. It is helpful to call to mind that people in power get to impose their own metaphors. Those that were shaped in and by the family of origin need not be the ones that you choose for yourself when you have become your own person.

There is movement in my life, albeit very slowly, to find new meanings. Many of the new meanings are shaped by a feminist awareness of myself as a person who deserves to be nurtured by others, is capable of more than stereotyped behaviors, and enjoys exercise. When my husband and children do a substantial amount of the cooking, I now see them as nurturing me and not as them kicking me out of "my" kitchen. I see caregiving as changing; the competent nurse is not just broad shoulders and a maternal demeanor, but a professional capable of organizing complicated systems and doing research to improve patient care. I can appreciate how much I loved my mother and grandmother without making their health problems part of my destiny. I, who never participated in a regular exercise program until I was well into my fourth decade, now lament what chlorine does to a bathing suit, rather than muttering about how I look in a bathing suit.

This period of journal keeping put me in touch with the range of thoughts and feelings I had about being fat. I learned to go beyond society's "narrow" thinking about the fat and to appreciate the extent to which I was a "woman of substance" in the most complicated sense of that phrase. There was something freeing about using the journal to get in touch with the strength of character which made me want to be larger than the life traditionally available to women. In the process, I saw my fat as making sense and being positive. It represented my unwillingness to be the "little woman" while being true to the value system of my ethnic background.

As I explored these themes, I became very angry at our "you can never be either too rich or too thin" society which no longer particularly values heartiness, generosity, and nuturance. I was torn between being true to myself and being concerned about the stress being fat had placed on my heart and my joints. I wanted to take better care of myself, and at the same time not repudiate my "substance."

Seven years later, I have improved my diet (switching from a diet high in processed foods, salt, sugar, and fat to one relatively rich in complex carbohydrates, roughage, calcium, and iron) and my endurance (exercising at my local "Y" as often as my schedule permits). I have also joined the National Association to Aid Fat Americans (NAAFA) and regularly read the magazines geared to providing fat women with fashion and health tips—*BBW* (Big Beautiful Woman) and *Radiance*—because I want to take steps to value myself as I am instead of living the postponed life waiting for some Cinderella transformation. Through the journal, I was able to appreciate some of the major influences on my life, which helped me take control of what I am and want to be. The journal did not transform my life, but set in motion a full assessment of my situation which has led over time to behavioral change. I make healthier choices.

REFERENCES

Ernsberger, P., & Haskew, P. (1987). Health benefits of obesity. *The Journal of Obesity and Weight Reduction*, *6*, 69-81.

Keller, E.F. (1982). Feminism and science. *Signs: Journal of Women in Culture and Society*, *7*, 589-602.

Lakoff, G., & Johnson, M. (1980). *Metaphors we live by*. Chicago: The University of Chicago Press.

MacKinnon, C.A. (1982). Feminism, Marxism, method, and the state: An agenda for theory. *Signs: Journal of Women in Culture and Society*, *7*, 515-544.

Moffat, M.J., & Painter, C. (Eds.) (1974). *Revelations: Diaries of women*. New York: Random House.

Schwartz, S.H., & Inbar-Saban, N. (1988). Value self-confrontation as a method to aid in weight loss. *Journal of Personality and Social Psychology*, *54*, 396-404.